ACU-YOGA

ACU-YOGA

Self Help Techniques to Relieve Tension

MICHAEL REED GACH
with
CAROLYN MARCO

HEALTH 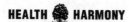 HARMONY

An imprint of

B. Jain Publishers (P) Ltd.

An ISO 9001 : 2000 Certified Company
USA — Europe — India

ACU-YOGA

First Edition: July 1981
14th Printing: March 1997
Reprint Edition: 2000, 2003, 2006, 2009

Originally published by Japan Publicationns, Inc., Tokyo and New York

Published by Kuldeep Jain for

HEALTH **HARMONY**

An imprint of
B. JAIN PUBLISHERS (P) LTD.
An ISO 9001 : 2000 Certified Company
1921/10, Chuna Mandi, Paharganj, New Delhi 110 055 (INDIA)
Tel.: 91-11-2358 0800, 2358 1100, 2358 1300, 2358 3100
Fax: 91-11-2358 0471 • *Email:* info@bjain.com
Website: **www.bjainbooks.com**

Printed in India by
J.J. Offset Printers

ISBN 817021828-4

This book is dedicated to
The people who want to learn
Effective, natural ways that contribute
To their well-being and
The well-being of all humanity.

Preface

With the fast pace of modern living, people need ways to release stress more than ever before. *Acu-Yoga* is a powerful, practical tool that people can easily learn and use to relieve their stresses and tensions, and replace them with energy and vibrant health.

Look around you and see how most of us deal with stress nowadays. Mostly what we do is avoid it or try to suppress it by overeating, smoking, drinking or using over-the-counter medications or other drugs. Of course, all of these only compound the problem.

I know that people want to feel good, to feel healthy, to have ample energy throughout the day. *Acu-Yoga* can provide that. It can help us get back in touch with ourselves and our bodies. It can enable us to break the negative habits we have acquired and replace them with positive ones that support our health and well-being.

Many physical disorders such as headaches or backaches are either caused by or worsened by tension. We have the ability to turn these "minor" ailments around, to actively work toward health. *Acu-Yoga* is a health practice that can benefit many physical disorders, especially problems that involve muscular constriction.

Acu-Yoga is written to serve people with a wide range and variety of experience, from beginners to health teachers and practitioners. Its aim is to show the interconnections between the ancient practices of Yoga and the traditional systems of Acupressure. It is written as a self-help manual. The first section of the book discusses the origins and basic principles of *Acu-Yoga*. The second section contains four exercise series that can be used for daily practice. The last section covers twenty four common disorders that are related to stress and tension. Each section deals with the causes and gives practical self Acupressure techniques.

Many people are not familiar with Acupressure and Yoga. But both techniques are easy to learn and do. It's as simple as learning where and how to hold a point on a tight muscle, how to stretch and loosen it up.

Now that Yoga is demonstrated on national television and Acupressure is used by athletic trainers in national and international sporting events, more people are becoming aware of these ancient practices. This book was written to give people in all walks of life concrete, practical, and simple ways for helping themselves.

This book is not meant to take the place of Yoga or Acupressure instructors. Rather, *Acu-Yoga* complements classes in these health arts. By combining learning and practicing on your own with the personal attention and instruction of a good teacher, you can do more than with either approach by itself.

I sincerely hope that people try these techniques, practice them, and integrate them into · their lives. *Acu-Yoga*, a natural, easy form of self-care, can make a difference in your life, in how you feel every day. I am grateful for the opportunity to show what I have learned and developed.

MICHAEL REED GACH

If you have an acute or chronic disease, please seek medical attention from a qualified doctor. Although Acu-Yoga is beneficial in numerous cases, it is not a means of diagnosis or treating pathological conditions. Acu-Yoga can be used as an adjunct to a doctor's care, not as a substitute for medical treatment.

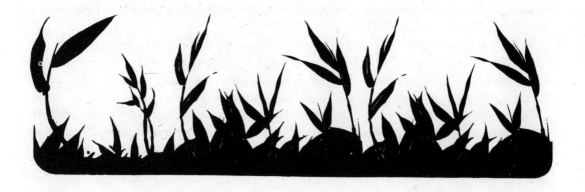

Acknowledgments

The development of *Acu-Yoga* is based upon centuries of practice and research in the Orient. *Acu-Yoga* also could not have developed into a form of physical therapy without the valuable ancient teachings that were passed down from generation to generation.

I am forever grateful for the guidance and wealth of information given to me by my Acupressure teachers, Ron and Iona Teeguarden, who taught me the depths of practicing Jin Shin Acupressure. Ron's encouragement inspired me to write this book. Iona's diligent research, substantial correlations, and organizational talents have been tremendous contributions. I wish to acknowledge the Teeguardens for teaching me Acupressure and the traditional principles of health maintenance.

Gratitude goes to Gurucharan Singh Fowlis, M. S. for initially training me to teach Yoga. His knowledge of yogic therapeutics inspired me to study the profound connections between holistic health systems. In understanding that his knowledge and high spirit is linked with the infinite chain of teachers who have transmitted the teachings of Yoga, I want to not only thank him but thank all gurus and yogis who channeled their inner wisdom and light into Yoga.

I especially wish to thank Carolyn Marco for organizing, editing, and rewriting the manuscript. Her knowledge of both Acupressure and Yoga and her writing skills have totally transformed this book into a comprehensive whole. I want to acknowledge Christel Busch R. N. for her illustrations and Andrew Partos and James Lerager for their photography. I want to thank Sylvia Quigley and Neeltje De Haan for modeling the postures and for their support. This book and cover were graphically designed by Ma Anand Zeno, also known as Diana Coleman. I can't express how grateful I am for her contribution. I also wish to thank Mary Tasch, Ph.D. and Ashoka (Michael Davis) for reviewing the manuscript from a yogic perspective; Paula Margolis, Nancy Iswomon and Kyle Suen for their advice and paste up work; Michele Petti and Wendy Warren for organizing and typing the manuscript; Sharon Schufman R.N. and Paul Warshow for helping me write parts of this material; and Josh Barron, Linda Gach Ray, Greg Hastings and Ana Vertel for their advice, consultation, and encouragement.

I acknowledge that it was the talent and contributions of women that transformed this book. I know that this book would not be what it is without their skills and creativity.

I especially want to thank Mr. Iwao Yoshizaki for selecting to publish *Acu-Yoga* and for giving the manuscript his personal attention. I wish to express my deepest gratitude to all the people at Japan Publications, Inc. who worked on producing and printing *Acu-Yoga*. I hope that the quality of this book will stand as an example of the value that can be generated when the resources of two great countries work together.

I could not have written *Acu-Yoga* without the compassion of all my teachers and the support of my family and friends. I wish to thank my Aunt Mitzi, who first introduced me to Yoga. My mother and father deserve the greatest acknowledgment for their guidance and for the years of love and affection that will continue to serve as a strong foundation in my life.

MICHAEL REED GACH

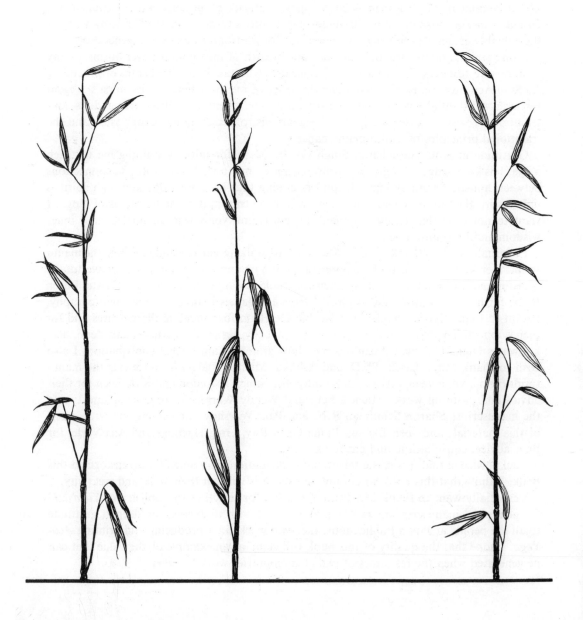

Contents

SECTION I:

An Introduction to Acu-Yoga

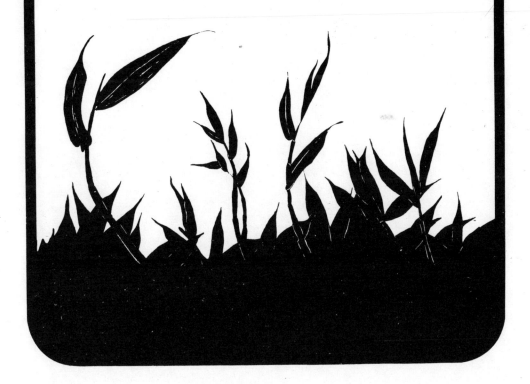

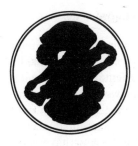

Chapter 1

The Background of Acu-Yoga

Holistic Health*

Acu-Yoga is a system of exercises that integrates the knowledge of two ancient holistic methods of health maintenance, Acupressure and Yoga. Increased effectiveness results from combining these two complementary practices of self-treatment.

Both systems relax muscular tension and balance the vital life forces of the body. Yoga does this through controlling the breath while holding the body in certain postures. Acupressure does this by directly manipulating body energy through a system of points and meridians. The pathways that the vital energy flows through are the meridians, and the points are the places where you can tap into that energy.**

In Yogic terms this vital life force or energy is called *prana*. Acupressure uses the Chinese name of *chi* or the Japanese term *ki*.

When tension accumulates around the points it blocks the energy from flowing properly, thus creating an excess of energy in one area of the body and a deficiency in another. Each Acu-Yoga posture, however, naturally presses and stretches certain nerves, muscles, and Acupressure points, awakening the meridians and releasing the tension in the points so that the energy can circulate freely. This process balances the body as a whole, and also stimulates it to heal itself.

---

* Holistic health deals with all the aspects of a person as a whole: body, emotions, mind, and spirit as one, not as separate parts.

** It should be noted that Acupressure and Acupuncture are based on the same principles, meridians, and points. Therefore, the terms "Acupressure point" and "Acupressure meridian," as used throughout the book, are identical to those commonly known in terms of Acupuncture.

Ancient Forms of Preventive Health Care

Yoga and Acupressure and both important traditional forms of preventive health care. They effectively release tension and eliminate toxins, both of which imbalance the mechanisms of the body. In traditional Oriental health care it is said that disease is initially caused by tension and stress, or, in other words, by *dis-ease*. Before the symptoms of any particular ailment manifest, there will be tension and toxicity in some areas of the body. It is to our advantage to work on our physical imbalances when they are at the least developed stage, that is, before the tension and toxins have caused damage to the internal organs. Acu-Yoga enables us to eliminate these tensions at this early stage before they have developed into illnesses.

The great sages of the East were masters of preventive health care. They were able to determine imbalances through traditional diagnostic methods, and thus avoid sickness. They knew Acupressure, certain breathing exercises, and natural diets to balance out specific conditions; many of these techniques are contained in this book.

Note that these methods were most effectively used to maintain people's health and to prevent disease. Herbs and Acupuncture were used in more severe cases, and drugs and surgery were used only as a last resort. Many of the exercises that follow were traditionally considered to be the highest forms of preventive health care.

The Nature of Disease

Disease is not just a conglomeration of symptoms. Disease is a state of being. It is reinforced by what we do with our lives. In fact, according to traditional Chinese health care, it is a clear reflection of how we treat ourselves in relation to our environment. If this relationship is harmonious, we reflect health. If your life style is not in harmony with your own nature, then you will eventually reflect disease. Harmony is the most basic law of the body. Disease is an expression of disharmony.

Many of us have gone through incredible changes in the past several years. Even though our attitudes, values, and life styles may have changed, we still carry deep emotional stress within us from the past. These unfinished emotional experiences are manifested internally as physical blocks. We all have tension to some degree, especially in this era of rapid change and over-stimulation. Yet, tension itself can be a part of the process of change. As a sign of imbalance, it is expressing what needs to change to restore harmony in the body. The purpose of tension is to guide us. However, most of the time we aren't aware of, or don't listen to our inner voices. When these signals are avoided energy blocks accumulate.

Physical and Emotional Health

The body must be used in order to function properly, that is, to remain healthy, to develop, and to grow. Some people have practically stopped using their bodies. The availability of cars, television, and other machines has changed many peoples' life styles. Daily chores that formerly required physical exercise, such as chopping wood and washing clothes, are now eliminated through the use of gas and electricity. These modern conveniences create comforts which can result in an unhealthy under-use of the body. Also, more jobs these days require sitting at a desk rather than physical exertion. The result is that people have become more sedentary.

Health centers, doctors, and physical therapists all over the world recognize the importance of exercise for maintaining health. From an Acu-Yoga point of view, tension is a stagnation of the bodily flows: the nerves, meridians, lymphatic ducts, and blood vessels. Lack of exercise contributes significantly to this stagnation. Physical weakness, low resistance to disease, accumulated tension, and toxicity caused by poor diet, alcohol and drugs add to it as well.

Emotional repression also contributes to disease, in that all emotional stress is stored physically as tension in the body. The stress of past traumatic experiences, neurotic patterns, and of day-to-day living cause physical blockages. For example, anger, sadness, frustration, or worry due to pressure from personal, work, social, and environmental problems can cause physical imbalances. So can repressed feelings from the past. These blocked emotions, whether conscious or not, lock the homeostatic or natural balancing mechanisms of the body, restricting their proper functioning. Emotional and physical problems can block our growth as individuals in many ways. Physical and emotional health, however, create a strong foundation for developing and unfolding on all levels of our being: physically, emotionally, intellectually, and spiritually.

Towards Radiant Health

The energy that is released in Acu-Yoga flows through the meridians, nourishing all the internal organs and all the systems of the body. This energy is the source of all life, and its flow is the key to radiant health. It functions to regulate and balance the respiratory, digestive, endocrine, vascular, lymphatic, urogenital, and nervous systems. It also balances our emotions. Thus, Acu-Yoga works to effectively create a feeling of well-being. By doing the exercises contained in this book, and becoming aware of this subtle and powerful energy, you can take responsibility for your health and improve your condition on all levels. For, when our energy is circulating properly we feel alive, healthy, happy, and in peace and harmony with ourselves.

The Origins of Acu-Yoga

"The science of Yoga dates from the so-called prehistoric times, when man led a natural life and was not under the spell of modern civilization."[1]

Many of the ancient civilizations lived according to the cycles of nature. They did not have to deal with the complications of the modern world that we must face every day. Their life styles were relatively simple, and this simplicity allowed them to cultivate an inner awareness of themselves. Out of this awareness and experience the systems of Acupressure and Yoga gradually developed.

The Development of Acupressure

There are three ways in which Acupressure originated and developed into a complete art of reawakening health: instinctively, objectively, and subjectively.

Since the beginning of recorded history, human beings have been *instinctively* drawn to hold places on the body that are blocked, ache, or hurt. One immediately holds a sprain, burn, or bruise to help relieve excessive pain. If you place a hand on your forehead to clear your thoughts or hold your lower back, you are actually treating yourself with Acupressure. Children often instinctively demonstrate this impulse when they are hurt. This indicates that Acupressure is unconsciously being performed all the time.

"Man's original medical tool is his hand, which he has instinctively used in order to alleviate pain. Whenever he is struck, stung, or seized with cramps, he involuntarily puts his hand to the painful spot in order to protect it or to rub, knead, or massage it . . . . In China, it was obviously realized from very early on that massage not only helped to relieve pain, that is to say, that its effect was not merely local; it was also seen that the stimulation of certain areas of the skin could affect the internal organs. Experience over thousands of years associated remedial massage with the same acupuncture points and meridians . . . ."[2]

Throughout the ages, people have also *objectively* found the most effective ways to help themselves through trial and error. For example, a common ailment such as a stomachache can be relieved with Acupressure by pressing or massaging different abdominal areas found by trial and error. The following quotation also illustrates the development of Acupressure by objective methods:

"In the dawn of history when stones and arrows were the only implements of war, many soldiers wounded on the battlefield re-

---

[1] Swami Vishnudevenanda, *The Complete Illustrated Book of Yoga*, page 19.
[2] Stephan Palos, *The Chinese Art of Healing*, page 154.

> *ported that symptoms of disease that had plagued them for years had suddenly vanished. Naturally such strange occurrences baffled the physicians who could find no logical relationship between the trauma and the ensuing recovery of health. Finally after many years of meticulous observation it was concluded that certain illnesses could actually be cured by striking or piercing specific points on the surface of the body."[3]*

Other objective findings that people have commonly used are their own first hand folk remedies that have proved to be effective. These findings have been preserved and developed through the process of objective conceptualization and reasoning. Methods of massage found to be effective for thousands of years were eventually integrated with the points and principles of Acupuncture. The best classical references of Acupuncture as well as the conceptual teachings from Huang-ti and Ch'i-Po, traditional Chinese doctors, were systematically included in developing Acupressure treatments.

> *"In antique China, in times which can no longer be historically defined, it has been discovered that there are certain points on the body which, if pressed, punctured, or burned (heated), had a beneficial effect on certain ailments. Through the exchange and widening of experience more and more points were discovered, by means of which it was possible not only to alleviate pain but also to influence the functioning of certain internal organs. Traditional medical literature reveals that the number of such points on the body kept increasing with the passage of time . . . . New connections kept being discovered between the various points and the internal organs."[4]*

Acupressure also developed *subjectively* through Masters whose keen inner awareness was so highly developed, so finely tuned, that they could literally feel and see the energy points and meridians on themselves and others. Each Master developed unique treatment combinations. Some sages would integrate breathing meditations along with "mudras" (hand positions) to stimulate certain Acupressure points for improving a person's condition. Another sage, being an herbalist, might prescribe certain plants, teas, and herbal preparations to help balance a disorder.

This information evolved as it was passed on within a family or village from generation to generation. The Chinese people have practiced Acupressure in this way since ancient times as a common way of life to keep their loved ones well and happy. Historically, this is how Eastern folk medicine grew.

> *"The realm of (Western) medicine could profit from a closer scrutiny of some of the ancient Chinese healing methods. Much beneficial truth may be lodged within the concepts derived from the careful observation of patients and within all the wisdom that has*

---

[3] Dr. Stephan Thomas Chang, *The Complete Book of Acupuncture*, page 14.
[4] Stephan Palos, *The Chinese Art of Healing*, page 40.

been collected over millennia—whether handed down orally or in
meticulously painted characters."[5]

The Development of Yoga

Yoga, a system of breathing movements and postures that the great sages spontaneously practiced over six thousand years ago evolved out of the same instinctual, objective, and subjective modes as Acupressure. These sages lived in harmony with nature as animals do, but with a human intelligence and consciousness which enabled them to observe the workings of their own bodies. Their simple but fluid life style sensitized them to experience the energy that flows through all forms of life. Thus especially attuned, and clearly feeling the dynamics of the meridians and nerve fibers, they developed natural ways to manipulate and direct these energy channels. Their movements and breathing techniques were the original sources of Yogic practices.

Many different forms of movement developed, depending upon the variations in climatic conditions, the culture, body constitutions, life styles, and the natural forces of the land. Some movements looked like wild tribal dances, surrendering the body completely to the forces of the universe. Some danced like rivers flowing, as in Tai Ch'i. Others allowed their bodies to receive the life force by moving into natural postures where their bodies would lock and breathe deeply.

Yoga further evolved as a natural form of folk medicine. Breathing exercises were taught and used by practitioners and sages who deeply understood the therapeutic effects of Yoga poses for various diseases.

> *"Correct breathing is the basis of all exercises recommended in China for longevity, as well as for the cure of several diseases. As early as the fourth century* B.C., *the philosopher Chuang-tze (. . . 400–370* B.C.*) promulgated that men of great wisdom fetch their breath from deep inside and below, while ordinary men breathe with the larynx alone. In other words, men even then were aware of the great value of deep respiration.*
>
> *The principle purpose of Chinese gymnastic exercises, as is the purpose of the Indian Yoga practices, is to attain proper circulation of the blood, which in turn, will ensure emotional balance and stability. This stability is to lend the body resistance against illness and consequently grant a longer lile."*[6]

Recent Additions

The Oriental healing arts changed with the invention of the printing press. What was once a practice of direct experience evolved into a study, a discipline. Intuitive Acupressure and Acupuncture treatments were eventually charted. The herbal experiments of the sages

---

[5] Heinrich Wallnofer & Anna Von Rottauscher, *Chinese Folk Medicine*, page 161.
[6] Heinrich Wallnofer & Anna Von Rottauscher, *Op. Cit.*, page 139.

were formulated. Yogic practices naturally were also put into a form, making it easier to learn from a Master. These written discipline did have their drawbacks, however.

> *"Around the 17th century, scholars started writing commentaries (on different approaches to Yoga) using logic instead of intuition."*[7]

And yet it is precisely this formulation of written materials that has made it possible for Yoga and Acupressure to spread around the world, in places far away from the cultures that developed them. This enables people in many varied places to benefit from these health practices who otherwise may never have known of them. At this point in history we are able to witness and experience a blossoming of the expansion and expression of this exchange between East and West. We are privileged to be able to benefit from the wisdom of these ancient cultures.

The Different Schools of Yoga and Acupressure

In the course of their development over the centuries, several schools of Yoga, and also of Acupressure, have evolved. Being aware of these different perspectives and methods, and of how they interrelate, will add in your understanding and practice of Acu-Yoga.

The Paths of Yoga

There are different types of Yoga, all of which lead to the same goal: the union of mind, body, and spirit. Each path is distinguished by particular practices, although the types of Yoga do overlap, merge, and complement each other.

Form of Yoga	Area of Concentration	Benefit
Acu-Yoga	Points and meridians	Increases circulation of the life energy
Bhakti Yoga	Devotion and love	Emotional development
Gnana Yoga	Knowledge	Intellectual development
Hatha Yoga	Postures and movement	Stretching and toning of the body
Karma Yoga	Service and action	Righteousness in living
Kundalini Yoga	Spinal column	Strengthening and balancing of the nervous system
Laya Yoga	Sound vibrations (mantras)	Strengthening and balancing of the endocrine system
Pranayama	Breathing	Strengthening and balancing of the respiratory system
Raja Yoga	Meditation	Mental mastery
Sahaj Yoga	Surrender	Spiritual purification

[7] Desai, *The Complete Practice Manual of Yoga*, Page 13.

Each of these forms of Yoga has a unique focus, and each gains strength from that focus. Each form of Yoga is also naturally interconnected with the others. These Yogic paths are linked together just as each system of the human body is linked together, forming a whole. When you improve the condition of one system, the whole body benefits. For example, if the respiratory system is improved through Pranayama breathing exercises, the whole body will naturally also be strengthened by the improved circulation that results. Although each form of Yoga emphasizes a particular approach to self-development, and has a separate identity and unique practices, each blends into the others.

Hatha Yoga, for instance, not only involves physical postures, but also breathing techniques and deep relaxation which complement the postures. Many people who practice Hatha Yoga naturally are involved in Bhakti and Karma Yoga. As one opens the body through Hatha Yoga it becomes natural to love and devote oneself to serving humanity.

Acu-Yoga gains its effectiveness by utilizing all paths of Yoga. Graceful movements, stretches, breathing exercises, postures, mudras,* sounds, visualizations, and meditations are used to awaken the life energy through the points and meridians. The combinations of techniques for self development are endless.

Acu-Yoga not only combines different types of Yogic practices but utilizes various forms of Acupressure as well.

The Types of Acupressure

There are currently four main types of Acupressure being used. Each form is distinct, yet they are also related, as is the case with Yoga. They are all methods using finger pressure to stimulate and balance the points and meridians, and can be done both on others and for oneself.

> **Shiatsu** is the most widely known. It uses finger (*shi*) pressure (*atsu*) on a series of points, pressing each one for three to five seconds, and can be somewhat vigorous.
>
> **Acupressure First Aid** is a more symptomatic approach, the knowledge of specific points being used to give temporary relief.
>
> **Acucises & Dō-In** are forms of self-acupressure that include self-massage of muscles and points, stretching, and breathing exercises.
>
> **Jin Shin** uses prolonged finger pressure on key acupuncture points to balance the meridians and functions of the body. At least two points are held together at the same time. Jin Shin promotes emotional stability and reawakens the joy of living.

We live in a time when many disciplines, many techniques, and many teachers are available. Each of us has to learn how to balance between the opportunities, to either focus on only one discipline for many years, or to study a number of techniques at the same time.

---

* Mudras are Acu-Yoga postures that produce electrical currents through the meridians.

Historically, people would follow the discipline of their Master, whom they loved and respected. These people committed themselves to one method which they studied and practiced in depth. They were forbidden to change the traditional teachings that they learned from their Master. From their focussed devotion they received the maximum benefits of the discipline. The danger in this, however, is in becoming closed or fanatical. Even when people practice with love and enthusiasm, they can sometimes tend to cling to what they know as a form of security, especially if they have chosen to accept only one method.

Acu-Yoga, which brings together many approaches and techniques into a holistic unification, has its own set of pitfalls. When you expand yourself to gain breadth as well as depth, opening up to many pathways, sometimes you don't know which way to go. If you know many exercises with different variations, and a number of breathing techniques, hand positions, and points to hold, you could possibly tend to get scattered by trying to learn or do too much at once. In practicing this holistic integration, it is important to focus yourself to gain the full benefits. For example, concentrating on a few postures, points, and breathing exercises until you master them is more beneficial than doing many different techniques incompletely. With a balance of focussed and expansive thinking and practice, you can unfold an infinite amount of energy through the exercises of Acu-Yoga.

Going Further: Acu-Yoga

Although Acupressure was developed in China and Yoga stems from India, both originated similarly from the depths of human awareness. It is from these primal origins of Acupressure and Yoga that Acu-Yoga was developed. Its roots extend into the source of creation, into those infinite universal energies that once moved people in harmony with the forces of nature.

Both of these traditional forms of practice further evolved into disciplines for study. These two great self-healing teachings of the Far East could never have been correlated without the wisdom of the ancient sages and the dedication of the practitioners and teachers who passed on the knowledge from generation to generation.

The challenge of evolving Acu-Yoga further lies in the hands of the New Age people for developing both the intuitive and intellectual aspects of this holistic health practice.

The Philosophy of Acu-Yoga

Acu-Yoga reflects the intuitive holistic philosophies of Yoga and Acupressure from the ancient cultures of India and China. These philosophies stem from direct experience. People who practice Yoga and Acupressure in depth are in touch with the inner mechanisms of their bodies. Their beliefs are derived from subjective experiences, from an inner assurance of truth. Western philosophies, on the other hand, take the opposite approach of being based on logical theories, with very rational premises. Intellectual concepts define and dominate a Western philosopher's outlook. Eastern belief systems, however, are grounded in awareness.

Types of Awareness

There are three main types of awareness: physical, emotional, and imaginative (mental awareness, or fantasy). Our physical awareness is composed of our gross sense perceptions of hearing, seeing, touching, smelling, and tasting. Our emotions are more subtle, inner parts of our being. Our minds reflect yet another state of consciousness, where we can receive intuitive information, and project it through inner voices, visual images, or extra-sensory perceptions. Our minds can also analytically and logically organize our knowledge and experiences.

These three levels of awareness overlap, directly affecting each other. (In the following diagram, this is represented by the shaded areas.) For example, a headache or stomachache, seemingly physical ailments, can often cause depression, or an emotionally low feeling.

Similarly, physical illnesses can block our mental faculties and imagination, and cause

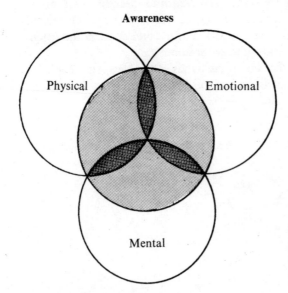

Spiritual awareness, the innermost core of our being (represented by the center circle), develops when these three functions are in harmony.

us to emphasize the negative aspects of things. Conversely, our thoughts are powerful, and if we think negatively we can limit or even harm ourselves physically and emotionally.

These three faculties, however, can also work together positively to create a more complete health or balance in us. When we feel good physically, it is easier to feel good emotionally and to have a positive mental outlook. Also, through visualization we can use our minds to help balance our bodies and emotions. And when we feel happy, it benefits us both physically and mentally. Acu-Yoga functions to help create positiveness on all three levels by integrating them into a healthy, working whole.

The Philosophy of Oneness

As expressed in the diagram above, the most important concept and experience of Acu-Yoga is the realization that ultimately all things are one. In other words, everything is interrelated to, and connected with everything else. We are not separate from our environment, but are part of a great unity that includes the tiniest atomic particle and the largest galaxy. To realize the interconnection of all things is a wondrous feeling. It is the experience of infinity, of the source of all life, energy, creativity, and truths.

Oneness can be experienced through the practice of Acu-Yoga which opens up the Organ Meridians and the Great Regulatory Channels. Acu-Yoga works directly to release blockages in the points, releasing energy into all the meridians for clearing the body and mind. This process frees the person so that he or she can experience inner peace. All existence becomes unified as one. The experience of oneness encompasses all consciousness as these great channels flow through the body.

The Tao: An Oriental Symbol of Unity

The Chinese call universal consciousness the Tao, or the Way of Nature. The Tao is the symbol of the infinite. It is boundless, encompassing the interactions in the universe on all levels: celestial, planetary, seasonal, historical, national, personal, chemical, anatomical, biological, geological, astrological, etc., beyond the limitations of time and space.

The Tao is a state of consciousness. It can be achieved through Acu-Yoga and meditation, where all things come together as one whole integrated unit. Life is this way. All forms of matter are in motion, vibrating constantly at varying speeds. Everything is constantly changing and interacting with everything else. From galaxies to molecules, everything moves in cycles, weaving together in a cosmic dance. In India, this reality is called "lila," meaning universal play.

The Tao includes everything in the universe, and "Yoga" means union. Taoist Yoga, therefore, is a way of living that unifies all realms of existence. A Taoist way of life is not just a set of spiritual exercises, but a way of manifesting oneself in harmony with life through meditation, thought, and action.

Yin and Yang

The world is constantly changing. The continual changes in all the elements of creation are an expression of the interplay between two basic polarities. *The Yellow Emperor's Classic of*

25

Internal Medicine* refers to these dual forces as yin and yang. These two primal elements interact as complementary opposites, and are illustrated by the following symbol.

 This yin-yang symbol represents the most important universal laws of change. It tells us that there are opposite elements that form a whole, and that things exist in relation to their opposite. Also, one changes into the other at its extremes. Night and day, winter and summer, cold and heat, receptivity and activity, femininity and masculinity, respectively, are some yin-yang relationships.

The dots in the center of these two elements indicate that some of each element is in the other. In other worlds, nothing is solely yin or yang, black or white. There are always shades of gray. For instance, there are some female qualities in men and some male qualities in women.

In human nature, there is a tendency to take things that are relative as absolutes. Culturally, we are trained to see things as either good or bad. These judgments keep us from experiencing the world as it is in the here and now. Yin and yang cannot be categorized as either good or bad. It's a dynamic principle of the way things change and is a description, not a judgment. Judgments are based on separations, while the interaction of yin and yang embraces unity.

Through the dynamic and fluid interaction of these forces life energy is created, generating the vibration referred to as Ki, Chi, or Pranic energy. Ki energy is concentrated in the living cells of plants and animals. The Ki energy of inorganic matter such as metal, however, is more condensed, more frozen or firm, but exists nonetheless.

> *"According to Yoga philosophy, there is no lifeless matter, for everything is consciousness itself. Scientists tell us that inside the tiniest particles of atoms is incredible movement. If there is movement, there must be some kind of energy to cause it, and that energy is the basis of all life."*[8]

The focus of Acu-Yoga is on this energy level. Practice develops that quality of awareness of Ki energy, which is the key for growth, creativity, and love. Acu-Yoga reunites the polarities of the yin and yang within the human body into one harmonious vibration. This unity enables the consciousness to expand from the finite to the infinite self, shifting into a level of energy awareness whose nature is harmony, balance, and flow.

The Law of Karma

Once you experience the principle of oneness, you ean easily see how one thing affects the other. If everything is interconnected, then any change will affect everything else. It is a law of nature. The law of karma states that everything that happens in the world affects you. It also means, on the other hand, that everything you do affects the whole world. It is inspiring to think of being so interrelated, considering the overwhelming apathy and alienation that pervades in this age. We have the ability to change the world by changing ourselves. The unfolding of Karma is a slow but powerful process of life.

---

* An ancient Chinese medical text written over four thousand years ago.
[8] Swami Vishnudevenanda, *The Complete Illustrated Book of Yoga*, page 6.

The law of Karma relates to all relationships like a mirror reflects an image. Karma means consequence. Everything you do has its consequences. If you avoid certain people, others will certainly avoid you. If you are selfish, you will eventually find yourself in a shell of indulgence. You cannot escape what you do in life.

If, on the other hand, you treat yourself with love and respect, you will be loved and respected. If you see the universe as one perfect entity, the world will show you how perfect it really is. If you love, you will be loved. It is a Karmic law that if you give, you shall receive. Why worry about your life? Everything is merely a reflection. You cannot be cheated. It all comes back eventually, because in the end it is all one. You cannot even take "short cuts," because everything you do has a consequence. Relax, just be yourself. Trust and have faith in the balance and harmony of life.

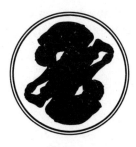

Chapter 2

Basic Principles of Acu-Yoga

Discipline

To attain any goal, discipline is necessary. In Acu-Yoga our goal is self-evolution, and some self-discipline is needed to keep us working toward it. When you first start to do Acu-Yoga you may feel stiff and not be able to stretch very far. You may experience some difficulty in the postures, in controlling the breath, and in quieting the mind. It is especially important at this stage to use your discipline, and try to do some Acu-Yoga every day, even if it's only for ten or fifteen minutes. After you've been practicing for a while, however, you will probably find that you won't need as much discipline to keep up, because it becomes enjoyable to do!

You might also want to make a calendar chart that you can check off when you do your Acu-Yoga exercises. This, or any other method that works for you to acknowledge yourself, can sometimes give you that last ounce of motivation to keep practicing.

After two or three weeks you will notice a difference in your body. You will feel more limber, and may move more gracefully. As you continue, you will develop better muscle tone, and possibly lose some inches from your waist. The spine will become realigned, improving the posture and nervous system. Circulation will improve, slowing the heartbeat and balancing blood pressure. You may start to gain new realizations about yourself. During the deep relaxation that follows the exercises, you may experience moments of inner tranquility. The energy channels, or meridians, of the body will start to open. The potential amount of Ki energy in your body will increase through the practice of the postures, deep breathing, and the stimulation of the points and meridians.

An understanding of the basic principles of Acu-Yoga, including discipline, will enable you to get more out of the practice that you do on your own, and will help you to create your own individual patterns of exercises. Be sure to familiarize yourself with this material before going on to the sets of Acu-Yoga exercises.

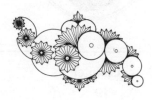

Body Awareness

In order to participate in life as fully as possible, you must cultivate awareness, and learn to know yourself. Body awareness is an important foundation for the practice of Acu-Yoga. Your body is constantly sending out a flow of thoughts and feelings which are messages for you to receive and act upon. For instance, when your shoulders become tense, it's a signal to change. You might need to get away from what you are doing, or from your immediate environment. You may only need to change the position of your body, or just taking a deep breath might relax your shoulders. If you can attune yourself to the inner mechanisms of the body, then you will be practicing Acu-Yoga in daily life.

The development of body awareness includes the following elements:
- Intuition
- Mental Attitudes
- Physical Awareness
- Centering Meditation
- Balancing Pain and the Emotions through the Breath
- Awareness in Daily Life

Trusting Your Intuition

You can cultivate an understanding of your own inner voice. In Acu-Yoga this communication with your inner self is called "the teacher within." The teacher within is the most valuable source of constant information and wisdom for knowing yourself. It is the most profound teacher you will ever find in terms of learning about yourself and receiving inner guidance.

If you know yourself on all levels, you are better equipped to handle any situation. If you know your intentions in any given moment, you can respond more directly and effectively. It is also important to know the condition of your body. If you know where you are stiff, and you know exercises for stretching out that part of the body, then your awareness of that stiffness becomes a clue for you to act upon. If you are aware that your inner voices are clues to guide you, and you act upon your intuitive thoughts, then you will be your own teacher and will grow at an amazing pace.

While practicing Acu-Yoga you will learn about yourself. The thoughts that arise during Acu-Yoga exercises may result in clearer insights about yourself. As a body therapy, Acu-Yoga opens a constant flow of messages from the teacher within you. It strengthens your growth potential by developing an awareness of the inner mechanisms of the body. This self awareness enables you to utilize your body for being most effective in the world.

By consciously practicing with an awareness of your body, you can gain more strength and personal power. The first step is to trust yourself. This trust of your own feelings, responses, actions, needs, etc., forms a foundation for all other relationships in life. The more you experience these relationships with an open mind, the more you will be able to trust and respond openly and clearly. Through the practice of Acu-Yoga, you can gain a new sense of yourself by listening to the teacher within for meaning and guidance.

Mental Attitudes

Your attitude about doing Acu-Yoga (or anything else!) strongly affects what you are doing. Check out what your attitude is. A negative or judgmental attitude can hinder your experience by blocking off the positive aspects that surround you. When you let go of that rigidity or negativity, you can regain a clarity in the present moment. In the here and now you can discover many things, especially when you are practicing the exercises of Acu-Yoga and are tuning into the messages of your body.

A wide range of attitudes may surface while doing Acu-Yoga. There are two extremes to this range. One is negative, where it becomes a drag. It's frustrating when you are stiff, and really do not want to do it. But there is also a positive attitude where it is fun, when it is a joy and a challenge to move and stretch. With a positive attitude you can go deeper and deeper inside yourself. Close your eyes so that you are not distracted, and pay closer attention to what you are feeling.

The "will to become" is an important drive for practicing Yoga as well as for improving the quality of one's life. It enables you to contact the place within you where you want to become more, you want to stretch more, you want to live a deeper, fuller life. Develop this kind of attitude as you practice the exercises in this book. Put your heart into whatever you do.

Physical Awareness

Every position in Acu-Yoga stimulates and affects different systems of the body. Each posture or pose influences certain endocrine glands, nerves, muscles, organs, and meridians. Even when you're not doing Acu-Yoga, the posture of your body relates to how you feel, and is an expression of what your body needs. Becoming aware of how you carry your body is an important goal in Acu-Yoga. This awareness not only enhances the effectiveness of Acu-Yoga, but of all your pursuits in life.

There is a process that you go through with each exercise. When you first learn a new exercise it is just a technique. This is the first stage of grasping the mechanical aspects of the exercise. From a set of mechanical techniques, the exercise becomes a more refined movement, smooth and graceful like a dance. In this second stage you still have to concentrate on the mechanics of the exercise, but at the same time you can become more aware of yourself through the dynamics of the movement. The third stage progressively develops as you begin to master the exercise or pose. At this point, the exercise becomes a meditation where you no longer have to concentrate on what you are doing, but can feel the energy and totally experience the entire movement.

Always tune into your body when you practice the exercises. This is best accomplished by simply closing your eyes, and turning your attention to the feelings in your body. Do the exercises without strain. Let your body stretch as far as it wants to go, trusting your own judgment. In practicing it is essential to trust your own limitations. Remember that your pace will vary, depending on the circumstances at any particular time. Be flexible and recognize that you will discover the pace that's right for you. We are all individuals, and have different needs and abilities. There's no competition in Acu-Yoga.

Acu-Yoga is an art of relieving tension. Instinctively, we use our hands to hold areas where there is pain and pressure, to help release the knots of tension which collect around the Acupressure points. Actually, this is how you locate the points: by feeling for and holding the places where you are tight. Often it is important to hold these points during or after an exercise in order to help release that area. In practicing the exercises, you can learn to adjust your hands and body weight and hold the blocked areas. Once you are directly on the tense area and your body position is comfortable, patiently keep your body still for a minute. In this way you can deeply but gently work on releasing your tensions.

Many times after you do an Acu-Yoga posture, you may get lightheaded, or feel new sensations moving through your body. This is what happens when the Acupressure points begin to release. The energy that was bound up as tension inside the point is now able to circulate throughout the body. This is the most important time to let yourself deeply relax, in order to allow for the distribution of the released energy. Through the development of an awareness of your body by cleaning the mind and tuning into the Acupressure points and channels, the path of Acu-Yoga unfolds.

Learning to Center

Centering the body physically in daily life is another one of the fundamental aspects for developing body awareness. It is a way to bring all parts of yourself together. In Acu-Yoga, centering means feeling at home with yourself, comfortably relaxed, and in touch. Centering in daily life means being clear and grounded in the world. The following meditation is a tool for learning how to achieve balance, peace, and tranquility through centering.

Prayer Pose Meditation

In a sitting position, place your palms together up against your chest, at the center of the sternum, and close your eyes. There is an Acupressure point there, Conception Vessel 17, which may bring out a warm feeling inside your heart. It is located on a bony protrusion of the sternum in between the breasts at the level of the heart. It is the most centering point of the body, and is called the "Sea of Tranquility." Concentrate on breathing into this point. Stay in contact with your breath, keeping the eyes closed. Let yourself breathe long and deep into the chest for a few minutes.

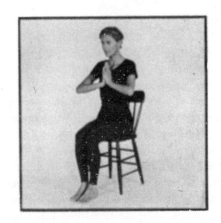

Balancing Pain and the Emotions through the Breath

If you push yourself too far, you will reach a point where an exercise may become painful. What you want to do is stretch to the point where you feel some degree of both pain and pleasure. If you only feel pain doing an exercise it indicates that you are pushing yourself too hard. You should release a little so that you still feel the stretch, but the position is comfortable. Always focus on your breath when you do feel pain. Imagine you are breathing into and out of the painful stretch. Long, deep breathing is a key for opening up tightness in the nerves and muscles.

The breath is the key to self-awareness. When your breath is shallow, you do not really have control of your emotions or identity. If you increase the capacity of your breath, making it long, deep, and gentle, you can gain full awareness of yourself. But many times, when some part of you is blocked, it is difficult to breathe fully. It might be due to a number of things: constriction in the chest due to emotional pain or anxiety; a great deal of grief or sadness; holding on to an unfulfilled expectation; or it might be due to a physical disability. Whatever the cause may be, difficult breathing relates to some kind of blockage. The purpose of tuning into your body is to discover the inner language of these body expressions. The more aware you can become of yourself, all parts of yourself, the more alive you will be to experience the wonders in life.

The greatest Yogis in India developed their inner awareness to a high degree through their Yoga practice. They were able to feel each system, each organ, the flow of each vessel, meridian, and nerve. Some were able to control their blood flow, heartbeat, and other physical phenomena. These Yogic Masteres were also able to direct their vital energies in the meridians through advanced meditations based on body awareness. You can master your own body through Acu-Yoga. The first step is to make contact with yourself and feel which parts of your body are blocked. Concentrate on sending your breath into those places. This will help to release the constriction so that the proper fluids and energy can flow through to these areas.

Awareness in Daily Life

A special beauty of Acu-Yoga comes in applying it in your daily life. You don't have to do Acu-Yoga strictly in a regimented, scheduled way. These techniques can be used spontaneously, whenever you want or need them, at any time. At work, for example, you may discover through your growing awareness that the way you hold your body creates tension. You can then use Acu-Yoga points and stretches to undo the blockages, and learn new ways of sitting or standing that don't cause tension.

If you go jogging or running, you can use Acu-Yoga to stretch your legs and help deepen your breathing. If you get cramps or gas while running, Acu-Yoga can also work to relieve any pain and tension.

At all sorts of odd times, such as when watching TV or movies, talking on the phone, reading, or even when waiting in line, you can use Acu-Yoga! You can practice deep breathing, you can hold points, you can improve your posture, and you can stretch tight, tired muscles. Have fun creatively integrating Acu-Yoga into your daily life.

Body awareness unfolds as a way of centering, grounding, and as a way of attending to or loving yourself. All aspects of your life are contained in the inner worlds of your body. It is important to know the language of the body, to know how it expresses itself. Listen to what is going on inside your body and pay attention to all of its expressions. The breath, posture, various symptoms, emotions, and tensions are all messages and inner teachings that constantly come from within. To develop this sensitivity is a life long, day to day challenge.

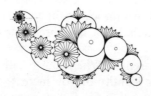

The Flexibility of the Spine

The spinal column is the foundation of the body. The nerves that go to all parts of our body and to all our internal organs branch out from the spinal cord, which is located inside the bony vertebral column, or spine. There are Acupressure points related to all of the internal organs and functions located along the spine. Therefore, when any vertebra is out of position, it affects the nerves and muscles in the local area, and also the internal organs associated with it through the related nerves and meridians. Muscular tension will collect around the imbalanced area, and can ultimately cause back pain, and more severe back problems. By systematically stretching your spine in all directions, however, you can release these tensions and help keep your spine properly aligned.

There are two very important principles regarding the flexibility of the spine. Firstly, it must be stretched in all its six possible directions: bending forward, backward, to each side, and twisting to each side. This creates a balance and a symmetry in the spinal column. Secondly, when you do an exercise that stretches the spine in any one direction, be sure to follow it with one that stretches it equally in the opposite direction. In other words, after you do one pose, do a counter-pose as a complementary balance. The plow pose, example, curves the spine forward. To balance this pose you would do the cobra pose, which curves the spine backwards. When you create your sets of Acu-Yoga exercises for yourself, be sure to follow these principles in order to work in the most complete and balanced manner possible.

The Acu-Yoga postures work on all the various parts of the spine. The cobra pose, for example, works on the lumbar vertebrae of the lower back. A variation on the same pose, however, can be effective for blockages in the upper back. The traditional postures work on all segments of the spine, from the sacrum at the base of the spine to the topmost cervical vertebra upon which the skull rests.

Basic stretches should be practiced first to prepare the body for the more difficult and complex poses. Two fundamental stretches should be done before you go on to any others. First take a couple of minutes to stretch out the sciatic nerves which run down the backs of the legs from the sacroiliac region. The sciatic nerve is sometimes called the "life nerve." It is one of the largest nerves in the body, and is therefore capable of transmitting much Ki, or life energy. Stretching it is the most fundamental exercise in Acu-Yoga, and daily practice promotes longevity. Once you master this, all the other postures become much easier.

Secondly, the spinal flexes are basic exercises which are different from most of the others in that instead of holding the stretches, they involve movement of the spine back and forth, and twisting to each side. Health and beauty are contingent upon the flexibility of the spine. If your spine is flexible and in alignment, the result can be seen in your whole body. If you have a limber spine you will have a youthful body; stiffness in the spine is a sign of aging. Beauty is a reflection of inner harmony and good health. Parts of the body not regularly used tend to contract as you grow older, and this rigidity is a slow form of atrophy. If a person, however, is well-balanced, gets enough exercise, and has a harmonious lifestyle, he or she will glow with the naturally beautiful inner radiance of vibrancy and health.

Breathing Techniques

The breath is the most profound tool known for purifying and revitalizing the body. Something as basic as the breath reflects how you feel about yourself, as well as how you relate to the world. If your breath is shallow, all of your body's vital systems will be functioning at a minimum level. If your breath is long and deep, however, the respiratory system can function fully and properly, and oxygenation of the body cells will be complete.

There is a close correlation between the physiology of the breath and the psychology of behavior, since the way you feel physically affects how you feel emotionally, and how you interact in the world. Because breathing is a key to physical well-being, or to the lack of it, it has a large part to play in determining how we feel emotionally from day to day.

According to traditional Chinese physiology, the human potential lies with the kidneys, which were thought to be the body's energy storage tanks. The Chinese invented deep breathing exercises to charge these organs with vital energy. Deep breathing increases both the amount of fully oxygenated red blood cells, and the release of the waste product, carbon dioxide, which chemically changes into carbonic acid if not eliminated through proper respiration. Accumulated carbonic acid must be filtered by the kidneys, and this taxes the body's essential energy, "Ching Chi," which the ancient Taoist sages worked to develop. Since Ching Chi can be developed through the breath, and is passed on, being inherited by each offspring, it points to the potential of human evolution.

The following are the five main breathing techniques used in Acu-Yoga:

Long Deep Breathing is the most basic technique for balancing the meridian pathways, the endocrine system, and the emotions. Inhale deeply into the abdomen, the diaphragm, and finally into the chest. Hold the breath for a few seconds, then exhale slowly. Consciously breathe smoothly, gradually, and deeply, concentrating on making each breath full and complete.

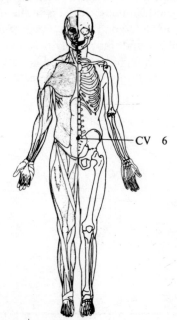

CV 6

Hara Breathing nourishes the internal organs, giving the body power and endurance. The *Hara* is a vital energy center located three fingers width below the navel, at the Acupressure point Conception Vessel 6. Concentrate at this point while breathing deeply into the lower abdomen. Let your belly come out as you inhale. Feel the breath being expanded into the depths of the belly. Exhale, drawing the belly in, letting the energy circulate throughout the body. Directing the breath through the "Sea of Energy," as the *Hara* is called, strengthens the general condition of the body.

Breath Visualizations tap the infinite creativity of the mind by focussing on certain parts of the body. With the breath, the potential for self-directed actualization and healing expands. Breath visualizations use the power of the imagination to unblock areas of the body, promoting new awareness, positive attitudes, and a greater circulation of Ki energy. There are endless variations and possibilities for visualizations, the one chosen being determined by the individual's condition, and the particular situation that the person wishes to affect. Different combinations of color, sound, body parts, guided meditations, and physical, mental, and emotional affirmations help to channel the power of the breath. The following is an example of a simple visualization that helps "Breathe Away Your Tension."

> *Close your eyes, and focus on an area of your body that needs attention. Imagine that the breath is a substance that is penetrating into that area. Concentrate on breathing into the blockage. If the tension is in your neck, for example, breathe deeply in all those tight muscles. Hold the breath a couple of seconds at the top of the inhalation. Exhale, smoothly allowing your tension to let go. Use the breath as a tool for releasing stress. Inhale deeply, bringing the Ki energy into the affected area. Exhale, feeling this energy circulate throughout the entire body.*

Breath of Fire is a powerful Yogic technique used with the postures. It strengthens the nervous system, cleanses the blood, and expands the electro-magnetic field of the body. The Breath of Fire consists of short, rapid breathing through the nose (making about one breath per second), concentrating on pumping the breath *out* by contracting the abdomen. This technique also stimulates the nerves in the nasal passages, and charges the body with immediate energy.

Holding the Breath during a specific pose serves to massage different internal parts of the body. The blood pressure temporarily rises when the breath is held. Once you let go of the breath, the blood pressure goes down and stabilizes as internal stress is released, encouraging deep relaxation.

Meditation

One purpose of meditation is to transcend the usual limitations of human consciousness and expand to higher levels of awareness. This can be accomplished by focussing your mind, which allows you to temporarily step aside from its constant chatter. The mind can then go beyond its normal scope into a vastness that cannot be described, only experienced. This is because language is geared toward the physical and the tangible. It cannot describe where the sky ends, or the feeling of visualizing how many grains of sand there are on all the beaches and deserts of the world. The mind can only experience the totality of creation through the process of meditation.

Most people operate from a surface shell which is very limited in scope. They are totally identified with their egos and personalities, which are protected by this surface shell. They have not yet developed a sense of themselves beyond their personalities—that divine, eternal spark of unlimited awareness. The mind can become rigid, and closed off from its own magnificence, just as the body can become stiff and inflexible. As the body contracts, the mind develops layers of resistance, which become the limitations of human consciousness.

Meditation is a tool that enables us to go beyond these limitations. Like anything worthwhile, it requires effort and discipline to achieve success with it. The many benefits of personal and spiritual unfoldment that can be attained through this inner work are so rewarding that it becomes a joy, not a duty or an exercise. Whatever effort you do put into it comes back to you many, many times over, so that your life begins to expand in ways you had never imagined. Meditation unfolds this process of self-fulfillment.

The stillness achieved during meditation also slows down the metabolism of the body. This provides a deep state of rest which has great therapeutic benefits; it rejuvenates the entire body, especially the nervous system.

Some meditations concentrate on the breath, some on a sound (known as a "mantra"), and some focus the mind on the circulation of energy (Chi) or light throughout the body.

Meditative exercises that use sound, such as singing or chanting a word or phrase, vibrate the thyroid and parathyroid glands, stimulating them to secrete. They also activate the pituitary gland, which balances the endocrine system as a whole.

Concentration is meant to be effortless. Instead of struggling and fighting with the stream of thoughts, just keep your attention on the meditation. As thoughts float to the surface, let them come and go without trying to control them. Observe the flow of your thoughts, watching them come into your mind, and then letting go of them. When you notice that your attention has wandered, gently let go of your thought, and bring your awareness back to the meditation. It's this continual process of letting go that benefits the brain.

The Three Locks*

In Acu-Yoga meditation and exercises, three contracted positions, known as "locks," are used. They are the Root Lock, the Diaphragm Lock, and the Neck Lock. When you apply all three simultaneously, it is known as the Master Lock.

These locks channel energy, preventing it from dispersing by concentrating it on the various chakras (vital centers). The Root and Diaphragm Locks are used to reach the Acupressure points which lie internally in the abdominal region. The Neck Lock stimulates important Acupressure points in the throat and neck areas.

According to Yogic tradition, the application of these locks increases blood circulation, and helps regulate the endocrine glands and rebalance the reproductive system. Regular practice strengthens the urogenital organs, so that the occurrence of menstrual cramps in women and wet dreams in men can be reduced.

Each of these locks is used in meditation to channel energy through the meridians, stimulating a natural self-healing process.

Root Lock (*Mulabandha*)

This lock stimulates energy in the first and second chakras by contracting the rectum, sex organs, and navel. To perform Root Lock, take a deep breath, and as you exhale do the following: (1) draw the anal sphincter muscle in as if holding back a bowel movement; (2) contract the urethral tract as if holding back urination; and (3) pull the abdomen in towards the back.

Kundalini Yoga commonly uses Root Lock to rechannel dormant energy at the base of the spine up to the higher chakras for conscious, creative use. From an Acu-Yoga perspective, this powerful contraction unites the Yin and Yang meridians.

Diaphragm Lock (*Uddiyand Bandha*)

This lock releases physical constrictions in the third chakra by pulling the diaphragm up and in. To do Diaphragm Lock, take a deep breath, and after the exhalation pull the upper abdominal area up and in by strongly contracting it. This enables pent-up energy to connect with the Governing Vessel, the Great Central Channel of the spine. It also internally massages the muscles of the diaphragm and heart, works on the "middle warmer" of the Triple Warmer Meridian, and also stimulates the third and fourth chakras, which govern the respiratory and cardiovascular systems.

Neck Lock (*Jalandhara Bandha*)

This lock opens the energy to the upper chakras, and is an important position for all meditation. It elongates the cervical vertebrae, which promotes the flow of cerebrospinal fluid to the brain. It also allows the nerves and meridians to transmit the Chi, or vital energy, in the strong and balanced way characteristic of meditation. It especially stimulates the throat chakra, and the glands associated with it.

To do Neck Lock, sit with your head straight, and imagine that there is a wire connecting your chin and the hollow at the base of your throat between the collar bones. Now lift your chest and slowly move your chin along this imaginary wire, so that it is pointed

---

* One should receive personal instruction from an experienced Yoga teacher and practice these locks with care.

towards that hollow at the base of the throat. This stretches the cervical vertebrae into a straight line. Don't let your head fall forward, and don't *move* your neck. Simply let the head tilt downward so that the neck becomes stretched, and locks in this position.

Master Lock

This consists of simultaneously applying the Root, Diaphragm, and Neck Locks. Circulation through the Central Nervous System increases greatly during the practice of these locks, that is, they channel Kundalini energy up the spine. Activity in both the *Sushumana*, the central spinal nerve cord and the Governing Vessel (the central spinal meridian) is balanced.

> ". . . . *In the back are located all the nerve fibers that mediate movement. If the movement of the spinal nerves is brought to a standstill, the ego, with its restlessness, disappears as it were. When a man has thus become calm, he may turn to the outside world. He no longer only sees the struggle and tumult of individual beings, and therefore he has that true peace of mind which is needed for understanding the great laws of the universe and for acting in harmony with them. Whoever acts from these deep levels makes no mistakes.*"[9]

Meditative Exercises

For the first four exercises, sit in a comfortable position with your spine straight, either in a chair that supports your back, or in Lotus Pose, as described below.

Lotus Pose

Lotus Pose is the classic traditional posture for deep meditation. The legs cross at key Acupressure points* which stimulate the deep internal Ki to circulate throughout the brain, enhancing the meditation process.

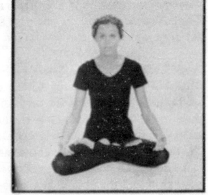

1. Sit with your legs straight in front, extended forward.
2. Spread your legs apart, into a "V" shape.
3. Bend your right leg, and place the top (instep) of the right foot on the upper left thigh.
4. Now bend the left leg and place the top of the left foot on the upper right thigh.

---

[9] Richard Wilhelm, *I Ching*, page 201.
* Spleen 6, Gall Bladder 39 and 40 are pressed in Lotus Pose. The feet also press Liver 10 and 11 on the inside of the thigh.

Exercise 1: Meditation for Internal Nourishment

1. Sit comfortably with the spine straight, and close your eyes.
2. Apply Neck Lock by lifting the chest and pressing the chin lightly into the hollow of the throat.
3. Connect the tips of the thumb and index finger of each hand, and rest the back of the hands on your knees.
4. Inhale deeply. Exhale, and at the end of the exhalation apply the Root and Diaphragm Locks for a few seconds by contracting your rectum, sex organs, abdomen, and diaphragm.
5. After a minute, discontinue the Root and Diaphragm Locks at the end of each exhalation. Simply meditate on breathing into the *Hara* (lower abdomen).
6. Continue for two more minutes. Be sure to keep your spine straight.

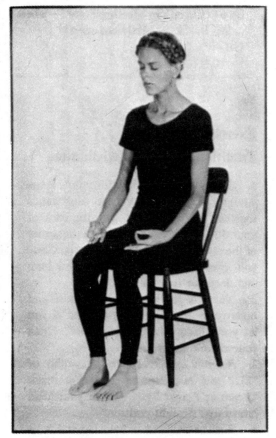

Focus on your breath. Gently control your respiratory system, making each breath grow longer and deeper.

Breathe out any tensions you feel restricting your lungs from moving fully and naturally. Feel your mind clear with each breath.

Notice the resistance your mind creates: the barriers of judgment and analyzing that it comes up against. Take several deep breaths and let go of the barriers. Breathe deeply and gently, as if you are breathing love in.

Hold the breath at the top of the exhalation, feeling its fullness. Exhale smoothly, feeling the goodness of the breath energy circulating throughout your body.

If you meditate on the breath in this way as much as possible it will increase your effectiveness in life. You can do it any time, even when you're occupied with your daily activities. Put your attention on your breath for a few moments and feel the benefits it provides.

Acu Points	Traditional Associations
Sp 6 ("Three Yin Meeting Place"—where the Sp, Lv, & K Meridians meet)	Menstrual problems; genitals
GB 40	Balances the Gall Bladder Meridian
Lv 10, 11	Menstrual irregularity

Exercise 2:
Traditional Healing Meditation

1. Sit comfortably with your spine straight. Place the palms of your hands together in Prayer Pose, with the back of your thumbs pressing up against the center of the chest at the level of the heart. Close your eyes, and let your breath grow long and deep for one minute.

2. Next, as you inhale, slowly raise and open your arms up over your head as you let your head slightly drop back. Open yourself to the universe.

3. As you exhale, chant the sound of "SU," and let your arms slowly float back to center, Prayer Pose, and let your head return to a straight position.

4. With your hands in your lap and your eyes closed, sit quietly with your spine straight, and imagine that you can still hear the sound vibrating. Discover the benefits of the exercise as you sit for a few minutes in a relaxed way.

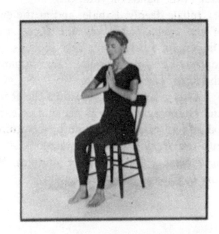

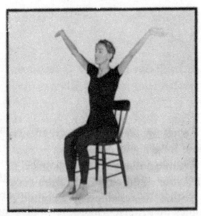

Exercise 3:   Waterfall Meditation

1. Sit comfortably with your spine straight, and close your eyes.

2. Place your palms over your ears so that your index and middle fingers touch the base of the skull (underneath the oc-cipital ridge, GB 20). The thumbs gently press the muscles on the sides of the neck, where the "windows of the sky" (p. 201) points are located.

3. Breathe long and deep. Listen to the inner sounds of the breath, and imagine a gigantic waterfall.

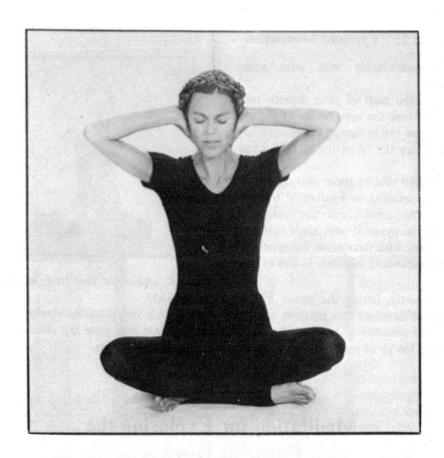

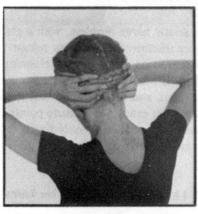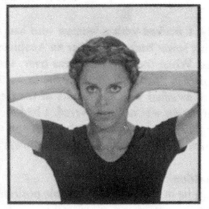

4. As you inhale, imagine that the water (representing Ki, or vital energy) rushes into your head. As you exhale, hear the water fall down your neck, shoulders, and chest, and into the abdominal organs, legs, feet, arms, and hands.

5. Continue to visualize the waterfall as you breathe deeply through your nose. Gently let your hands rest in your lap, and sit quietly for a few minutes.

Exercise 4: Pyramid Meditation

1. Sit comfortably with your spine straight.
2. Place the pads of your thumbs into the area where the upper ridge of the eye socket joins the bridge of the nose (Bladder 2). Place the fingertips of each hand together.
3. Let your elbows come slightly out to the sides, creating an equilateral triangle with your forearms. Close your eyes. Now visualize the pyramid or triangle that you are forming with your arms. Imagine this triangle expanding infinitely in size as you breathe.
4. Sit quietly, letting the power of the meditation increase. This position can attract great amounts of energy. There are no limits. Let go of your concepts. Empty

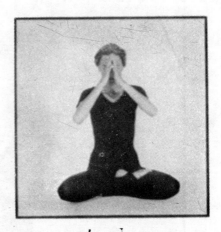

yourself, and allow your inner experience to expand.
5. After a few minutes, slowly let your hands come into your lap. Sit quietly to discover the benefits.

Meditation for Exploring the Cause of Disease

Recently, I worked with a woman who had a sciatic nerve problem, with a great deal of pain in her lower back. I gave her an Acupressure treatment designed to release this problem area. When the treatment was over, she moved her hips around, claiming that her condition was "better," and that she knew that "it wasn't going to go away overnight." I was not satisfied with the results of the treatment, and inwardly felt that the source of her sciatic pain was not uncovered. I had located the exact Acupressure points that were blocked and extremely sore for her, but the treatment seemed to only touch the surface. Consequently, I led her through the following meditation:

Body Position
> Sit or lie in the most comfortable position. I had her lie down with her knees bent and her feet on the floor, comfortably apart.

Hand Position "Mudra"
> Place the hands on the affected area. In this case she placed her hands on top of each other, palms down, underneath the sacrum (bony area at the base of the spine).

Breath
> Begin long, deep breathing with the eyes closed. Direct the breath mentally into the affected area. Become more aware of your body as you breathe.

Mentally

Let your mind go. Let go of judgments, worries, fears. Consciously release the tightness inside the brain. Open up your head, letting go of the boundaries inside your mind.

Meditation

Ask yourself these questions, and listen for a simple reply:
- What caused my disease? What caused me to get sick?
- What can I do to help my body heal itself?

Let your body be still; keep your eyes closed; let the breath be deep and even; and your mind will empty and open as you ask yourself these questions. The cause and natural cure will come to you if you truly want to know the answers.

After the guided meditation, my client's eyes were clear and full of light. She had a big smile on her face. "I got in touch with the parts of myself that were holding on to my mother. I realized that I internalized or unconsciously stored my hurt about her in my hips. You know," she said, still smiling, "She was really a pain in the ass!"

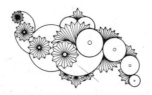

Deep Relaxation

Opening the Eight Regulatory Channels of Acupressure

The purpose of Acu-Yoga relaxation is to open the eight regulatory channels which serve to rebalance the body. The Acu-Yoga exercises work directly on all the points of the 12 organ meridians to release blocks of tension. This, however, is just half of the process of Acu-Yoga. When you go into a deep relaxation after these blockages are released and the body can completely let go, the eight extra or regulatory meridians become active. They serve as reservoirs, equalizing the streams of energy in the organ meridians. Their flow accomplishes this by channeling the excess Ki energy from areas that are too full into areas that are deficient. This is probably the most profound homeostatic mechanism of the human body, in terms of its ability to heal itself. This is also why relaxation is so important after doing Acu-Yoga, or after receiving an Acupressure treatment or other form of therapy or bodywork.

The last pose in a series of Acu-Yoga exercises should be done more strenuously to momentarily increase the blood pressure, work the muscles, and stimulate the nerves and meridians. This will facilitate a state of deep relaxation. Relax on your back with your eyes closed for ten to twenty minutes at the end of a series of exercises. Breathe long and deep into the *Hara* (the lower abdominal area), letting go of stress in all areas of the body and mind.

The whole consciousness changes during deep relaxation. There are no longer any physical (muscular) or mental resistances. The mind is able to go off into a far away realm, traveling in its consciousness, but also fully aware of the present. This deep state is called a "Yogic sleep," and just a few minutes of it has incredible healing powers. It completely refreshes the mental faculties, and revitalizes the physical capabilities of the body.

There are absolutely no dangers in doing Acu-Yoga if you use common sense and understand the principles of relaxation. The harder and longer you do an exercise, the more you need to relax. If you do these exercises and do not allow time to completely relax, then complications can occur. The exercises are very powerful, and the deep relaxation is a complementary balance just as important as the exercises themselves. Be sure to leave yourself plenty of time at the end of your sessions to gain the full benefits of this deeply relaxing and healing state.

Guidance for Deep Relaxation

> *After doing a set of exercises, lie down on your back, palms facing up. Close your eyes and feel your body relaxing. Wiggle your toes, letting them relax. Rotate your feet so that the ankles relax. Slightly move your legs, feeling your calves, knees, and thighs relax. Tighten your buttocks muscles and let them relax. Feel your sex organs and pelvis relax. Take several breaths into your abdominal area, letting your belly relax. Just let yourself relax. Whatever you are hanging on to inside your mind, just let it go . . . . Let your whole back relax. Relax your arms. Feel each finger relax. Tell your shoulders and neck to relax. Let go of your forehead and eyebrows. Let your temples and ears relax. Lips, teeth, and tongue . . . relax. Move your jaw from side to side, letting it relax. Relax your nose and your throat and tell your eyes to relax. Feel your whole body totally loose and relaxed.*

Deep relaxation comes by surrendering the mind. How is that accomplished? By letting go of all boundaries and barriers that are confining your mind. Let go of the attitudes and thoughts that create separations. Allow your thoughts to flow without trying to hang on to them. Just surrender, letting go of your judgments and expectations. Beyond all of these mental conflicts and restrictions are the infinite vibrations of the whole universe. This experience of oneness is one of the most important steps toward spiritual growth.

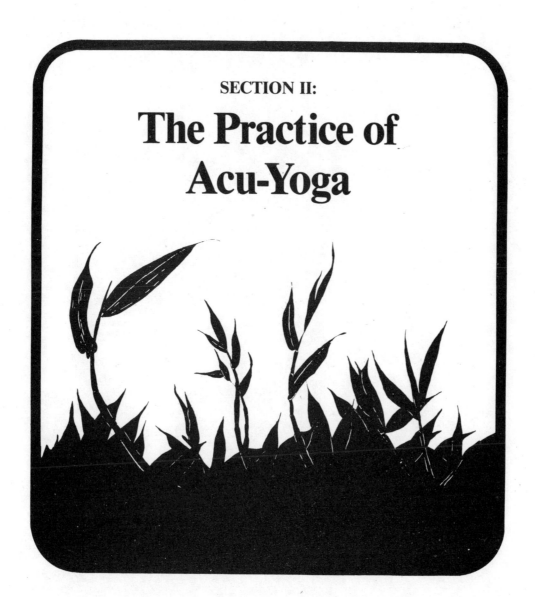

SECTION II:
The Practice of Acu-Yoga

Part A

Acu-Yoga Series of Exercises Based on Yoga

Introduction to the Practice of Acu-Yoga

Daily practice is the foundation of preventive health care. Consistent, daily routines, that stretch and strengthen all parts of the body enhance well-being. Unfortunately, many people develop the exact opposite: destructive habits that consistently imbalance and weaken the body, eventually contributing to various diseases. For example, smoking, drinking alcohol, and overeating are common ways people either escape from or temporarily release their stress. These habits, however, actually cause further tensions and imbalances in the body! However, these habits can be changed. We can choose to develop positive habits. We can consciously replace negative habits by cultivating healthful routines, or "positive addictions," such as exercise practices and healthier diets. In becoming used to these beneficial practices, we are developing habits that create and maintain radiant health.

This section of the book contains four complete sets of Acu-Yoga exercises, each with a different focus or approach. Each series of exercises is complete in itself and is designed to balance the body as a whole. Each set contains a progression of exercises that works on a different aspect of the body. The first two topics, "The Flexibility of the Spine" and "The Chakras," are based upon Yoga, and "The Regulating Channels" and "The Organ Meridians" have an Acupressure orientation.

Most of the important Acu-Yoga poses have more than one function or application, and are therefore purposely included in more than one section. This is why you will find that some of the poses are repeated in the various exercise sets.

Personal experience is the best way to discover which set of exercises best suits you. Choose one of these Acu-Yoga sets and practice it every day for one week. The next week choose a different set, and continue this way until you have done all four, noting how you feel during each one. At the end of the month, you will be able to choose which series best fits your needs.

Make your Acu-Yoga practice a habit by devoting about half an hour in the morning or the afternoon to your exercise routine. As you get past the resistances that may surface and learn to enjoy Acu-Yoga, your practice will become an essential daily activity that boosts your energy and well-being.

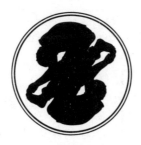

Chapter 3

A Whole-Body Self-Treatment
Emphasizing Flexibility of the Spine[*]

The spinal column holds a key position in the development of general health. Composed of 33 vertebrae, it encloses the spinal cord, which is made up of the nerves that stem from the brain. Each vertebra of the spinal column has openings through which the branches of these spinal cord nerves spread out, going to *every part* of the body.

The spinal column is also the principal structure for supporting the weight of the human body. When it is healthy and limber, it can function properly, and accomplish this easily. Poor posture and lack of movement, however, result in impaired flexibility. This can cause the spinal column to become weakened, and even pulled out of line by tension. Eventually, severe damage and deterioration can occur. We can prevent this degeneration through the practice of Acu-Yoga, the most outstanding system for developing and maintaining strength, flexibility, and balance in the spine.

People who practice Yoga have extraordinary spines. You can feel it if you've ever given a massage to some one who does Yoga as opposed to someone who doesn't. The vertebrae of a person who does Yoga are all very distinct and in line. The person who doesn't may have a great deal of chronic back tension. The vertebrae tend to be more difficult to feel due to the muscular armor or blockage. Acu-Yoga exercises can strengthen and relax the spinal muscles, harmonizing the whole vertebral column.

The following series of exercises energize almost all of the 31 pairs of spinal nerves which relate to every organ in the body. The series is designed to work from the base of the spine all the way up to the top, to promote flexibility and elasticity. By practicing these exercises, you can not only maintain good health, but reawaken a new awareness of life and vitality.

The way to increase the power of these exercises is to move with the breath, to establish

---

[*] Be sure to read the section "The Flexibility of the Spine" on page 34.

a rhythm that allows the muscles and nerves to relax. Breathe deeply into the stretch. The **power of the breath increases the effectiveness of the exercises.**

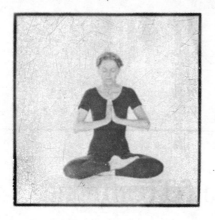

Breath Meditation

1. Sit comfortably, spine straight, with your palms together, against the center of your chest in prayer pose.
2. Close your eyes and focus on your inner awareness. Center yourself by feeling your breath grow long and deep.
3. Continue for two minutes, then take a deep breath and move on to the next exercise.

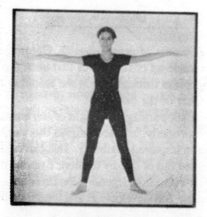

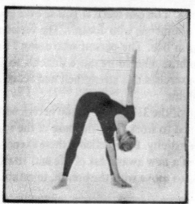

Cross Stretch

1. Stand with your legs about two or three feet apart.
2. Bring your arms out to the side, parallel with the floor and inhale.
3. Exhale, bringing the right hand toward the left knee, calf, ankle, or foot, depending on what is a comfortable stretch for you. Have your left hand stick straight up. Look at your left hand pointing straight up to the sky. Keep your legs straight.
4. Inhale and come back to the starting position.
5. Exhale, this time bringing the left hand to the right side, with your right hand pointing up. Look up at your right hand and stretch.
6. Continue for one minute, alternating sides.

Water Wheel

1. Stand comfortably with your feet about a foot apart. Put your palms against your lower back, fingertips by your spine.
2. Inhale and gently arch backwards, supporting your lower back with your hands.
3. Exhale dropping forward allowing your body to hang. Let your shoulders relax, droop and dangle.
4. Continue for one minute at your own pace, inhaling up and exhaling down. Feel the spine being flexed in both directions and your body weight as it shifts back and forth.

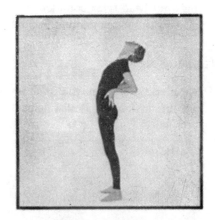

Traditionally these exercises have been used to develop sexual potency. They benefit the lower back region, and are also good for relieving pelvic tension. Once you get the rhythm, close your eyes and feel your pelvis pivot with the movement. Inhale and exhale through the nose, establishing your own pace of movement and breathing. Slowly increase the speed of the exercise with the rhythm of the breath.

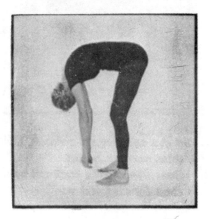

Cat-Cow

1. Get down on the floor on your hands and knees. Bring your head all the way up and arch your spine as you inhale.

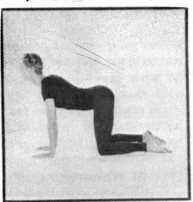
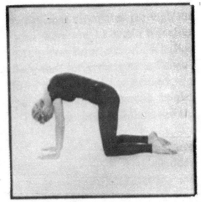

2.   Drop your head down and push your back upwards as you exhale. Relax your neck, letting your head relax completely.

3.   Continue for one minute, feeling your vertebrae flex in both directions.

Camel Ride

This exercise strengthens the spine in a way that aids in sitting straight for long periods of time in meditations. It also helps to develop the body's supply of stored energy.

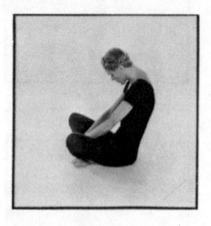 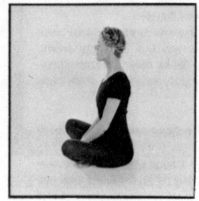

1.   Sit in a cross legged position, holding your shins near the ankles.

2.   Inhale arching your back and bringing your chest forward and up.

3.   Exhale as you lean back onto the coccyx bone (base of the spine) in a slumped position.

4.   Continue for one minute, breathing through your nose, inhaling forward and exhaling back. Keep your head relatively stationary as the lower spine flexes in both directions. Let the movement be graceful, not jerky.

5.   To finish, inhale up and hold the breath. Center yourself with the eyes closed, spine straight. Let your breath come out very smoothly and sit quietly for a minute.

Life Nerve Stretch

1. Sit on the floor with your legs spread wide apart.
2. Grab hold of your shins where you get a comfortable stretch. Keep the backs of your knees on the floor, and your legs straight throughout the exercise.
3. Inhale, stretching up, straightening your spine. Lift your chest all the way up getting a nice deep breath.
4. Exhale, coming down towards the left, your head aiming at your left knee.
5. Inhale stretching up to the center again.
6. Exhale bringing the forehead down to the right, towards the right knee.
7. Continue for one minute. Establish a graceful but vigorous rhythm.

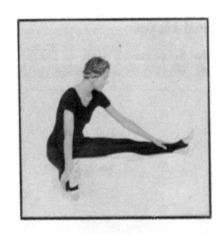

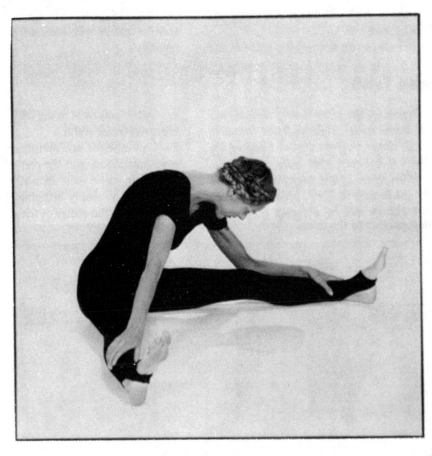

Spinal Flexes

Spinal flexes mainly work on the thoracic vertebrae, which are located in the mid-portion of the spine. It is beneficial for the liver, spleen, stomach, gall bladder, and pancreas.

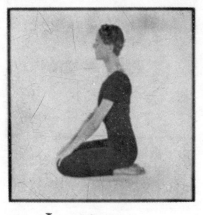 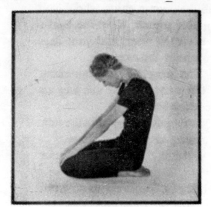

1. Kneel down and sit on your heels with your hands on your knees.
2. Inhale, arch the back, and raise the chest up and out.
3. Exhale as you slump your spine in the opposite direction.
4. Continue for one minute, slowly increasing the speed. The movement of this exercise alone will increase your breath capacity.

Spinal Twists

1. Kneel on the ground, and then spread your knees apart slightly. Your buttocks may be either on your feet or close to the ground in between your feet.
2. Place your hands on your shoulders with the fingers in front, thumbs in back. Your elbows will be pointing out to the sides, parallel to the floor.
3. Inhale and twist to the left, then exhale and twist to the right.
4. Continue for one minute, letting your head turn along with the rest of the body. Feel your spine twist in both directions.
5. Finish by firmly bringing your palms together into the center of the sternum and breathing deeply.

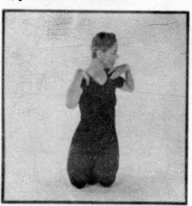 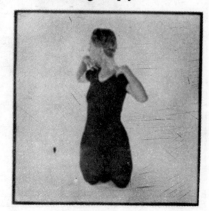

Yoga Mudra

This is a centering posture for generating love for yourself. One way to accomplish this is by breathing at a rhythm that makes you feel good. Breathing this way generates a healing tone or vibration throughout the body.

> *"Breath is the principal and essential power that can help in healing. There is a silent healing, and a healing by focussing the glance, touching it; but behind these different ways there is one power working, and that is the power of the breath. This power can be developed by physical exercises, by rhythmic exercises of the breath, by pure living and by concentration."*[10]

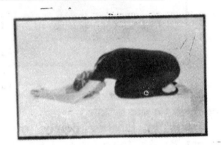

1. Kneel, and then bend forward, resting your forehead on the ground.
2. Stretch your arms out in front, bring your palms together, and let your forearms rest on the floor.
3. Let your body relax in this pose, for a couple of minutes, feeling your breath flow.

Stretch Pose

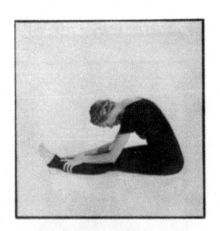

1. Sit on the floor and bring your legs out in front of you. Wiggle your feet, relaxing the joints in your knees and ankles. Let your body drop forward. Let your head come down and bob a little. Tell your head and neck to relax.
2. Grab hold of the shins or ankles, with your knees straight and your legs together.
3. Feel your breath. Let your body weight drop forward and down towards your legs, and begin long, deep, conscious breaths. With each inhalation, your thorax will raise just a fraction. The force of gravity will lower your body a couple of fractions each time you exhale. As you relax in this position, you will be able to come forward a little bit more with each breath without pushing yourself, simply letting gravity do the work.

4. Check your body out: make sure that your shoulders, neck, and head are completely relaxed. After one minute inhale and slowly come up into a sitting position.

---

[10] Sufi Inayat Khan, *The Book of Health*, page 52.

The Upper Back Flex

The last few exercises of this series work on the upper spine.

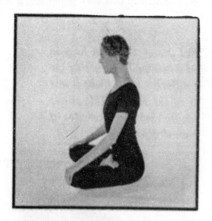

1. Sit cross legged again, as in the "Camel Ride," but this time hold your knees firmly, with your elbows straight.
2. Inhale and arch the chest up and out.
3. Exhale as you slump down and back, in the opposite direction.

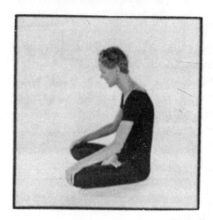

4. Continue to flex the spine in both directions for one minute.
5. Finish by inhaling deeply, sitting straight. Relax with your eyes closed for a minute.

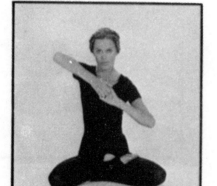

The Propeller

1. Sit cross legged. Cup your hands with your palms facing each other, and then bring them together so that your fingers lock together. Hold your hands this way at the center of the chest.

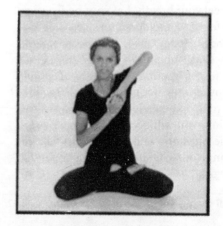

2. Inhale and bring your right elbow straight up, keeping your hands at the chest center.
3. Exhale as the left comes up.
4. Continue for one minute.

5. Inhale and bring your arms over the head, pulling outward against the interlock of your hands as you hold the breath in.

6. Exhale, relaxing your hands down. Gently shake your shoulders out and meditate on the circulation of energy in your body.

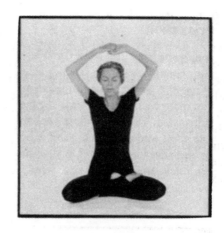

Shoulder Wings

This last exercise is for releasing tension in the shoulders. If parts of your body tingle or if you get light headed, as most people do, it indicates that more oxygen and nutrients are circulating into your brain.

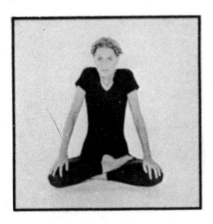

1. Sit comfortably cross legged and place your hands on your knees.

2. Inhale, and press your shoulders up toward your ears.

3. Exhale as they drop down and relax.

4. Close your eyes and put yourself into the breath as you continue the shoulder movements and breathing for one minute.

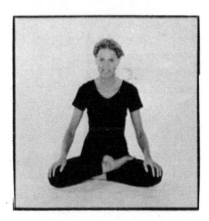

Deep Relaxation

Lie down on your back and relax for at least ten minutes. Let your hands be by your sides. Move your pelvis from side to side. Squeeze your buttocks and let them relax. Take several long deep breaths. Shake your shoulders and tell them to relax. Feel your feet, wiggle your toes and let them each relax. Rotate the feet at the ankles and tell them to relax. Feel your legs and hips relax. Tell your whole back to relax. Breathe deeply into your tummy, letting your whole chest and abdomen relax. Check out your fingers, letting each one relax. Let your arms and shoulders relax. Let your head roll effortlessly from side to side, feeling the whole neck relax. Breathe into your head, feeling your face and head relax. Just let yourself relax . . . .

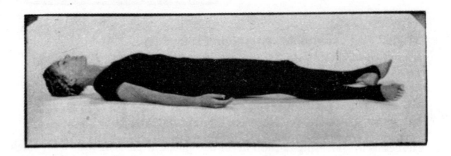

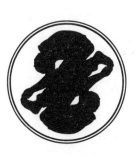

4 breaths per minute = balancing chakras

Chapter 4

The Chakras

The seven chakras are specific vital centers in the body that influence different aspects of our selves. They are energy vortexes that govern our physical, emotional, mental, and spiritual well-being. Therefore, they provide a foundation for the development of personal power.

All of the Acupressure meridians run through these centers and most of the pressure points relate specifically to one of the chakras. Many of the traditional associations of Acupressure points correspond to the characteristics of the nearest chakra. Since chakras are so related to Acupressure, being aware of them aids in one's understanding of the dynamics of Acu-Yoga.

From a neuro-physiological perspective, the chakras are represented as nerve plexuses from the spinal column and endocrine glands that connect with the internal organs. At the base of the spine is the first chakra, which is connected to the sacral plexus, the rectum, the prostate gland, and the male reproductive organs. The second chakra, below the navel, is related to the prostatic plexus, the adrenal glands, the female reproductive organs, and the kidneys. The third chakra is associated with the solar plexus, the spleen, the pancreas, the liver, and the gall bladder. The fourth is called the heart chakra. It is connected to the cardiac plexus, the thymus gland, and the pericardium. The fifth chakra relates to the thyroid gland at the level of the throat, which regulates the basal metabolism—the amount of energy used by the body at rest. The fifth chakra is connected by the vagus nerve and the cervical ganglion. The sixth chakra is associated with the pituitary gland, and the seventh chakra relates to the pineal gland.

Acu-Yoga uses the power of the breath to balance the chakras. In five minutes this can be accomplished by lengthening the respiratory process to four breaths per minute. These seven chakras are of central importance in Acu-Yoga practice. Each exercise works on a certain chakra, by flexing, stimulating, or stretching areas of the body. The following series of exercises works progressively from the first to the seventh chakra. By practicing this series of Yoga exercises you can systemically re-balance the energy in each of these vital centers.

Chakra	Acu Points	Location (Association)	Organs/Nerves Correspondences	Balanced Functioning: Emotional & Psychological Qualities	Imbalanced Functioning: Emotional & Psychological Qualities	Associated Physical Conditions
1st	GV 1, CV 1 GV 2, CV 2 GV 3, CV 3 Sp 12, 13 St 29, 30 Lv 12	Base of spine (Stability)	Sacral plexus Large Intestine Rectum Male reproductive organs Prostate	Security Stability	Self-indulgence Self-centeredness Insecurity Unstability Grief Depression	Hemorrhoids Constipation Sciatica Prostate problems
2nd	K 11, 12, 13 CV 3, 4, 5, 6, 7 GV 3, 4, 5 B 23, 24, 46, 47 GB 25	Mid-way between pubis & navel (Sexuality Creativity Energy storage)	Prostatic plexus Kidneys, Bladder Female reproductive system Adrenal glands	Patience Endurance Self-confidence Well-being	Frustration Attachment Anxiety Fear	Impotency Frigid Diabetes Over-sexed Kidney or Bladder problems
3rd	K 17, 18, 19 CV 10, 11, 12, 13	Between base of sternum & navel (Personal power)	Solar plexus Liver Gall Bladder Spleen Stomach Small Intestine	Personal power Self-motivation Decisions Willfullness Self-image	Powerlessness Greed Doubt Anger Guilt	Ulcers Jaundice Hepatitis Hypoglycemia Gall stones

	Points	Location	Plexus / Organs	Positive qualities	Negative qualities	Physical problems
4th	CV 17, 18 GV 10, 11, 12	Medially at the heart (Opens the heart)	Cardiac plexus Heart Pericardium Lungs Thymus gland	Compassion Acceptance Love Fulfillment	Insensitivity Emotionally closed Passivity Sadness	Cardio-vascular problems Arthritis Respiratory problems Stroke Hypertension
5th	St 9 B 10 CV 22, 23	Throat (Vocal expression)	Laryngeal plexus Cervical spine Thyroid gland	Communication Expression Creativity Interactions Inspiration	Stagnation Obsession Lack of expression	Sore throat Voice problems Thyroid gland problems Flu
6th	TW 4 GV 17, 18, 19, 24, 25 B 2	Third eye (Visualization)	Cavernous plexus Triple heater Gall Bladder Brain Pituitary gland	Intellectual & psychic abilities Visualization Imagination Projection Perception	Difficulty focussing in life Schizophrenia Detachment Intellectual stagnation	Headache Fuzzy thinking
7th	GV 16, 17, 18, 19, 20, 21	Top of head (Liberation)	Meridian plexus Liver, bladder Governing Vessel Gall Bladder Pineal gland	Universal energy & cosmic consciousness Cosmic love *Satori* Enlightenment	Depression Confinement Closed-mindedness Insanity Psychosis Worry	Cerebral tumors Cranial pressure

First Chakra

The first chakra is connected to survival, where the main motivation is to protect oneself as a separate being. Therefore, developing the first chakra means developing a sense of security in life. When you are insecure, you tend to cling to a love relationship, an occupation, a religion, or whatever. People who have trouble with their first chakra may not have developed a strong identity. They may not have found a purpose in their life. If they are too yin they might be ungrounded. If they are very yang they might be too attached to the material things around them, generally self-indulgent, or preoccupied with satisfying their own needs.

Here are two exercises that work on this energy center for developing stability, security, and balance.

Body Drops

This exercise works on Governing Vessel 1, an Acupressure point at the base of the spine.

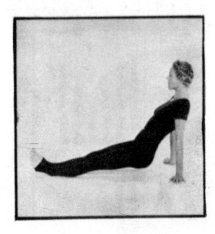

1. Sit on the floor with your legs stretched out in front of you.
2. Support yourself by placing your hands on the floor behind you.
3. Arch your buttocks up and bounce gently on the base of the spine.
4. Repeat step number three, eight times.

Stretch Pose (variation)

Traditionally, this pose has been used for conditions involving hemorrhoids, impotency, and constipation. It works on eliminatory energy. This exercise also stretches out the sciatic nerve, one of the largest nerves in the body, important for developing physical energy. Do the exercise on both sides, emphasizing the stretch on the tightest side.

1. Sit on the floor with your legs stretched out in front of you. Bend your right knee, and place your right heel between your genitals and your rectum. This puts pressure on Conception Vessel 1.
2. Your left leg remains straight out in

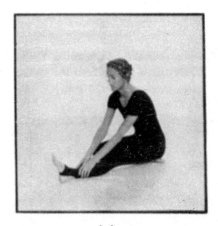 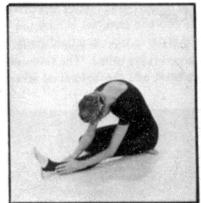

front of you. Grab hold of the left shin or ankle and inhale, straightening the spine.
3. Exhale, using your arm muscles to bring your forehead toward your left knee.
4. Continue for about a half minute on each side.

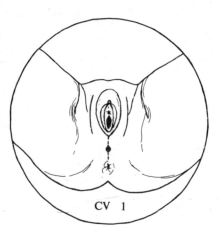

CV 1

Second Chakra

The second chakra governs our impulses of creativity and sexuality. If this chakra is too yin a person might have sexual problems, such as impotency. If it is too yang, sexuality can dominate one's life, so that sexual frustrations, thoughts, and fantasies are excessive. In either case, imbalances in the second chakra can lead to sexual problems.

In terms of other physical conditions, if the second chakra is too yin, then the abdominal area may be flabby, saggy, or generally weak. A person may also develop kidney or bladder weaknesses, and other urinary problems. If the second chakra is too yang, the muscles in the abdominal area will be constricted or tight and tension may accumulate in the lower back. The following exercises stretch and strengthen these areas to prevent such difficulties.

Cat-Cow

This exercise works on points along the spine, including Governing Vessel 3, 4, and 5. These points are called "The Gates of Life." Cat-Cow strengthens the second chakra, the lower back, and the abdominal area.

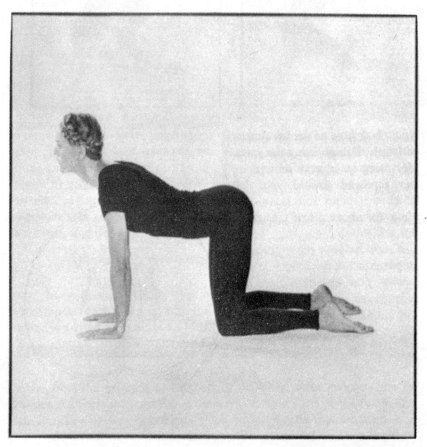

1. Get on the floor on your hands and knees.
2. Inhale, arch your back, and raise your head up.
3. Exhale, round your back, and let your head drop down. Your back curves upwards.
4. Establish a smooth rhythm of inhaling, head up, and exhaling, head down. Continue the exercise for about one minute.

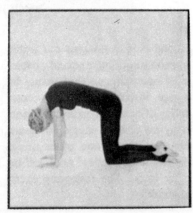

Locust Pose

This is an excellent pose for menstrual problems and for indigestion. In this pose Spleen 12, 13, Stomach 29 and 30 are stimulated. Please refer to the back of the section on "Pelvic Tensions" for an illustration of these points.

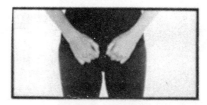
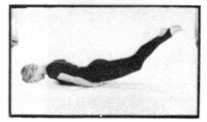

1. Lie on your stomach.
2. Make fists with your hands and place them under your groin area, with your chin or forehead resting on the floor.
3. With your feet together, inhale and raise your legs up off the ground. Begin breathing deeply with your legs stretched up for 30 to 60 seconds.
4. Then let your legs come down, rest your head on its side, and place your hands by your sides. Let yourself completely relax with your eyes closed, discovering the benefits.

Third Chakra

The third chakra is the power center of the body. If there is a deficiency (excess yin) in a person's third chakra, he or she may feel powerless. A person who is too yang, however, may have a tendency to be aggressive or greedy. The third chakra relates to the liver, gall bladder, stomach, and spleen. They help to regulate how centered we feel during the day in relation to our mental facilities and our ability to be self-motivated. Good diet (including green vegetables) and daily exercise (such as jogging or swimming) help to develop this chakra.

Pit Pose

This posture massages all the internal organs that are related to the third chakra, and is for developing a balanced sense of personal power. Each time you exhale you will feel a pressure on Stomach 22, 23, 24, Kidney 17, 18, 19, and Conception Vessel 10, 11, 12, and 13. The Pit Pose is one of the best Yogic exercises for releasing overall body tension.

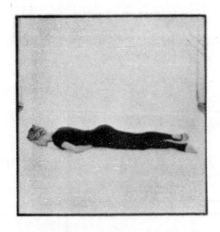

1. Remain lying on your stomach. Put your fists* underneath the rib cage into the area of your stomach, between the navel and the base of the breastbone. Begin breathing long and deep.
2. Press your navel point towards the ground and your breathing will internally massages the abdominal area.
3. After one minute, relax with your hands by your sides.

Spiral Flexes

This exercise flexes the spine in both directions. It works on the third chakra, and also affects the fourth chakra. This is an excellent exercise for emotional balancing.

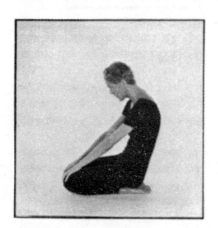

1. Sit on your heels with your hands on your knees. Slump down to curve your back.
2. Inhale, arch your back, and stretch your chest up and out.
3. Exhale as you slump down. Continue for one minute.

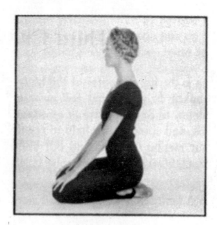

---

* If your fists create too much pressure and there is unbearable pain, place one hand over the other on the solar plexus area below your breastbone.

Fourth Chakra

The fourth chakra relates to our capacity to love, to open up our hearts, and to give. If the heart center is excessive (yang), then a person may be insensitive. If this chakra is deficient (yin), one may be hypersensitive, or feel emptiness within the heart cavity. When this chakra is blocked a person may appear to be cold, inhibited, or may exhibit passivity in his or her life. The fourth chakra governs joyfulness, and is the master control center for regulating the emotions. The following exercises benefit this chakra.

Flapping Wings

This exercise is helpful for constriction in the chest, difficulties in breathing, cardiac problems, and for reducing high blood pressure. The movement of this exercise stimulates the following points between the shoulder blades: Bladder 13, 14, 15, 16, 38, 39, 40. These points are traditionally used for cardiovascular problems.[11] Refer to the illustration on page 203.

1. Stand, bringing your arms up until they are parallel to the ground. Have your palms facing out.
2. Stretch your arms back without bending your elbows so you feel a pressure in the shoulder blades. Keep bending your hands backwards and feel the pressure in your wrists. Inhale, and raise your chest up and out.
3. Exhale, and keeping your arms straight, bring your palms together in front of you, curving the spine forward.
4. Continue to inhale as your hands go back and exhale as they come forward for one minute.

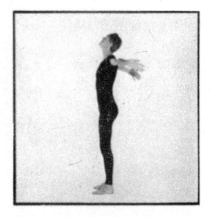

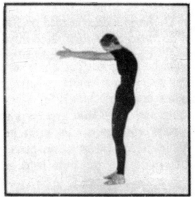

---

[11] Felix Mann, M. B., *The Treatment of Disease by Acupuncture*, pages 33, 37, 118, 172.

Cross My Heart Pose

This Acu-Yoga posture interconnects the first points of the heart meridian. In this posture, you can feel your heart beat.

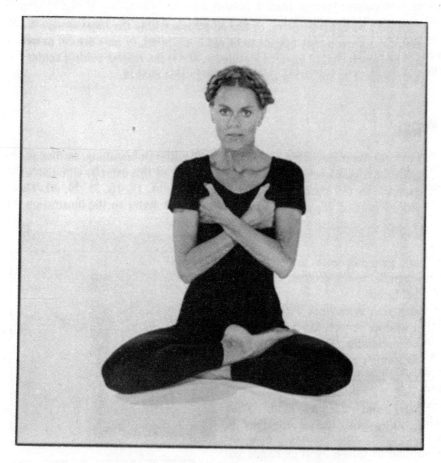

1. Sit in a cross-legged position with your spine straight.
2. Place your right hand in your left armpit and vice versa.
3. Close your eyes and feel your body. Meditate on your heart cave for a minute.

Calling to the Heart

The following exercise uses a sound to nourish the heart center.

1. Lie down comfortably on your back.
2. Close your eyes and allow your body to relax.
3. Inhale deeply.
4. Exhale, making the sound of "Yahh-mm."
5. Continue making the sound. Feel the vibration open up your heart cavity.

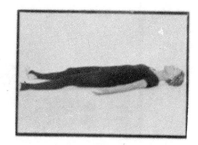

Fifth Chakra

The fifth chakra regulates sound. A person who talks very softly is apt to be more yin; a loud and boisterous voice represents a yang condition. Within the fifth chakra comes the power of communication and the ability of self-expression. Thus, difficulties in expressing oneself would demonstrate a block in the fifth chakra. Expressing what you want in life is very important. It makes the difference between being insecure and being in control, of being able to create your life. Opening the fifth chakra aids in this expression.

The following two exercises open up the points on the neck and stimulate the thyroid gland which is located in the cavity of the throat. The thyroid gland is important in regulating the amount of energy the body uses when at rest. It is also responsible for balancing the endocrine system which affects the internal organs and ultimately the whole body.

Side to Side

1. Lie comfortably on your back. Inhale deeply.
2. Exhale and slowly turn your head to the left.
3. Inhale as your head returns to the center.
4. Exhale as you turn your head to the right.
5. Continue the exercise for one minute, gently stretching the neck from side to side.

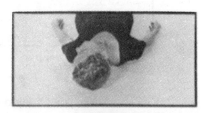

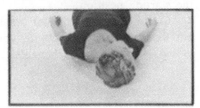

Bridge Pose

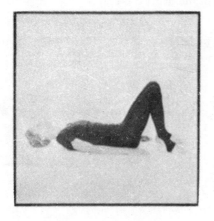

1. Lie comfortably on your back with your legs bent, the bottoms of your feet flat on the floor, and your hands by your sides.

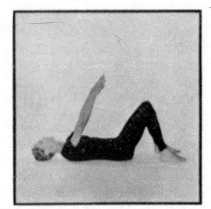

2. Inhale, bringing your arms up and back over your head to rest on the floor as you arch your pelvis upwards.

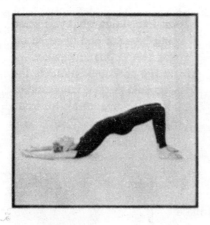

3. Exhale and lower your body down to the starting position.
4. Continue the exercise for one minute.
5. Relax on your back with your eyes closed, discovering the benefits.

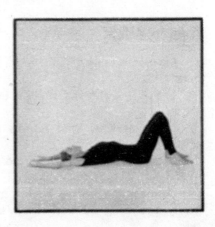

Shoulder Stand

Sore throats, speech problems, and neck tensions are also related to the fifth chakra. The shoulder stand works on shoulder tension as well. The hands support your lower back to strengthen the kidneys. This helps develop courage and self-expression.

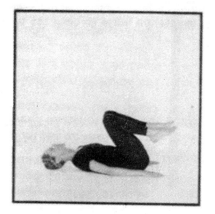

1. Lie down on your back. Inhale, and bend your knees toward your chest with your hands by your sides.

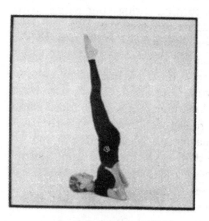

2. Exhale, and swing your legs back so that your hips come off the ground. Use your hands to support your lower back, with your legs bent over your head.

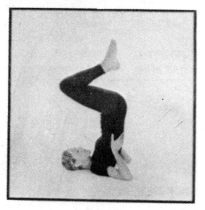

3. Move your hands towards the upper back as far as you can, straightening the back and legs.

4. Begin long, deep breathing. Breathing deeply in this position helps to stimulate the throat center.
5. Continue for one minute, and then come down slowly and rest, lying flat for a few minutes.

Sixth Chakra

The sixth chakra helps to develop a person's intellect. Blockage in the sixth chakra often manifests as a frontal headache, or as an inability to think clearly. These headaches, and scattered or confused thoughts may also be caused by blockages in the digestive system affecting this chakra. The following breathing meditation helps to clear the mind and strengthen the sixth chakra.

Clear Mind

This meditation works to stimulate the pituitary gland, the master endocrine gland, and to develop psychic abilities, your imagination, and your ability to visualize and project. The points affected are Governing Vessel 17, 18, 19, 24, and 25.

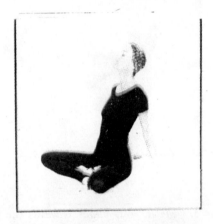

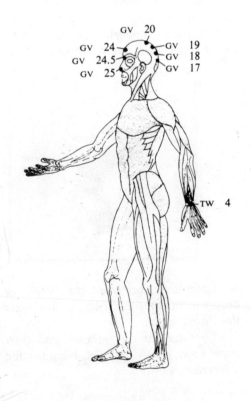

1. Come into a straight but comfortable sitting position. Bring your palms to the ground, six inches behind you with your fingers pointing away from you. In this position you should feel a pressure within your wrists (at the Triple Warmer 4).
2. Bring your head all the way back. Begin breathing deeply while focussing on the third eye (between the eyebrows).
3. Imagine the air is coming in and out of the third eye point. This stimulates the pituitary gland, lodged beneath the base of the nose just above the corners of the eyes.
4. Continue for one minute, then slowly return to a normal sitting position.

Seventh Chakra

The seventh chakra governs universal consciousness. When this center at the top of the head is opened there are no limitations in terms of time and space. The pineal gland, located in the center of the brain, is the core of this chakra.

Thousand Petalled Lotus Meditation

This breathing meditation stimulates the pineal gland, which controls one's ability to receive universal energy. The point at the top of the head (Governing Vessel 20) is called "the thousand petalled lotus." In China it is also referred to as "the hundred meeting place," since there are one hundred energies that flow up and meet here, at the top of the skull. Meditate on breathing deeply into this point. Let the breath penetrate Governing Vessel 20 as if a vortex of golden energy is descending into your body.

1. Sit comfortably and straighten the spine. Rest your hands on your knees, connecting the tips of your thumbs and index fingers. Open your eyes slightly and look at the tip of your nose.
2. Breathe through the nose in the following manner: Inhale four times, four short breaths one right after another, to the count of 1, 2, 3, 4. This meditation balances the relationship between the pineal and the pituitary glands.
3. Exhale slowly and smoothly. Continue to breathe deeply, gently, and quietly. Straighten your spine, visualizing a circulation of light throughout your entire body.
4. Close your eyes and roll them all the way up and back towards Governing Vessel 20 at the top of your head. Imagine that you are breathing into a window that opens into the top of your head.
5. Finish by relaxing on your back for a few minutes.

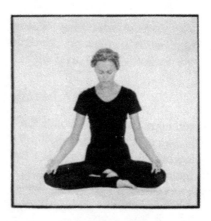

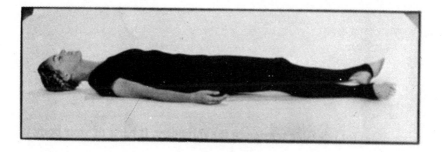

Acu-Yoga Series of Exercises Based on the Channels of Acupressure

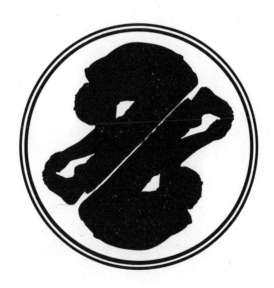

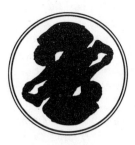

Chapter 5

The Eight Regulatory Channels

The Eight Regulatory Channels* function as the body's master homeostatic, or balancing mechanism. They harmonize all the internal organs and functions of the body. The doctors of traditional Chinese medicine said that these Channels work to balance the areas of excess blockage (yang, or hyperfunctioning), and the areas of deficiency (yin, or hypofunctioning).

> *"As early as the third or second century* B.C., *the* Book of Ailments *('Nan Ching') mentions the existence and importance of the special (regulating) meridians."*[12]

The Regulatory Channels of Acupressure are the foundation for Acu-Yoga therapeutics. Each of the traditional Yoga postures strongly stimulate these wondrous channels. Also, during the deep relaxation that follows the exercises, the Great Regulating Channels are reawakened to balance the whole body.

To understand the workings of these Channels, think of the twelve organ meridians as rivers flowing through the body, and the eight Regulating Channels are the lakes or reservoirs of energy which balance those rivers. The organ meridians flow continuously; the Regulatory Channels, their balancing system, only flow when necessary to normalize excesses and deficiencies.

Many of the key points from the twelve organ meridians that are used in Acu-Yoga lie along the Regulating Channels. These are especially powerful points because they are located where the eight Regulatory Channels and the organ meridians cross.

---

* Also known as the Extraordinary Flows, Strange Flows, Extra Meridians, or Special Meridians.
[12] Stephan Palos, *The Chinese Art of Healing*, pages 69–70.

Generally, these Great Regulatory Channels flow up the back and down the front of the body. Once an Acu-Yoga exercise is learned, students are encouraged to visualize the flow of the inner energies circulating through these miraculous Channels, as is taught in ancient Taoist Yoga meditations. The great Taoist sages pictured the energy forces flowing as water does, taking its natural course. It does not think about how to flow, it just follows natural laws.

> "[*Water*] *is in motion on earth in streams and rivers, giving rise to all life on earth .... It flows on and on, and merely fills up all the places through which it flows; it does not shrink from any dangerous spot nor from any plunge, and nothing can make it lose its own essential nature. It remains true to itself under all conditions.*"[13]

It is easy to see the similarity between water and human energy in the following quotation from the *Book of Changes* ("I Ching"). It shows how tension is caused, according to natural laws. The words in brackets have been added to demonstrate how these natural laws work in human energy systems.

> "*When water [Ki energy] in a kettle [body] hangs over fire [personal and social motivation/stress], the two elements stand in relation and thus generate energy [cf. the production of steam]. But the resulting tension demands caution. If the water boils over [meridian blockages causing physical illness], the fire [motivation/stress] is extinguished and its energy is lost. If the heat [work or effort] is too great, the water [Ki] evaporates into the air. These elements here brought into relation and thus generating energy are by nature hostile to each other. Only the most extreme caution can prevent damage.*"[14]

Thus, too much internal (personal) or external (social) tension damages our Ki, our life energy. Of course some amount of personal drive is necessary for a complete life, and there will always be societal tensions, but for health there has to be a balance between effort and stress, on the one hand, and rest and relaxation, on the other. Most of us are so strongly affected by these ever-present individual and social pressures, and yet we don't know how to properly balance them. We don't know how to put energy back into our systems, circulate or channel it fully, and then return a giving out flow to others. With our energy depleted, we become victims of tension and fatigue. We need to learn ways that enable us to not only compensate for what we lose from stress, but that go further to develop strong, vibrant health.

To achieve this radiant health, it is necessary to cultivate an awareness of how energy flows in the body as in all things of the world. The Chinese, living in harmony with nature, saw the interconnections of all things, and therefore made no separation between natural

---

[13] Richard Wilhelm and Cary Baynes, *I Ching*, page 115.
[14] Richard Wilhelm and Cary Baynes, *Op. Cit.*, page 245.

occurences and the dynamics of the human body. For thousands of years this ancient culture has studied the cycles of nature and the workings of natural laws in human physiology. The phases of the moon, for example, correspond with women's menstrual cycles. Times of day and night harmonize with human activity and repose.

Seasonal Changes

The changes of the seasons also affect our internal conditions and needs. We are part of nature, and therefore, are part of its changes. It is probably easier for us to be aware of the seasonal changes in plants and animals than in ourselves, but once we cultivate an awareness of these changes, we can feel how strong they really are.

The seasons maintain balance between growth and decay, between activity and rest. The life cycle of plants provides a clear illustration: during the spring tiny sprouts pop out of the earth, reaching their full maturity in the summer. The plant blossoms at its peak and turns to seed. It then drops its leaves and fruit in the autumn. The seeds become buried while the leaves are composted, enriching the soil. The seed lies dormant during the winter cold. The cycle of the plant is then ready to begin again as the seed awaits the spring to shoot above the ground.

We also have our seasonal cycles. Spring is the time of rebirth, of opening up to the new energies that burst out with the longer, warmer days. Summer is a time of activity and growth. Autumn is a time for calmness and reflection on the activities of summer. It is a time of harvesting or gathering in our Ki, which is stored or stabilized in the winter months of quiet and lessened activity. Then spring returns again with a new expansion of energy, to complete the cycle. By tuning into our breath, our bodies, and our energy meridians, we can evolve deeper and deeper into that feeling of connection and oneness with natural cycles, such as seasonal changes, and with all life.

Internal Balancing

When we open our minds and look at how the world works, we can see that the body has homeostatic mechanisms for balancing, just as nature does. Lodged inside the brain, the hypothalmus regulates body temperature. The thyroid gland, at the base of the throat, works to balance the rate of our metabolism at rest. The pituitary functions to regulate all of the endocrine glands. According to Chinese classics, the eight special Regulating Channels control all of these important self-regulating mechanisms of the body, which are necessary for maintaining health.[15]

Acu-Yoga enables us to stimulate the flow of energy through the Great Regulatory Channels. It involves learning to move and breathe in harmony, to be in balance with ourselves and our environment. These harmonious movements allow us to fully relax and recharge ourselves. The circulation is further enhanced by mental visualization, which work to direct energy along these special meridians.

---

[15] Refer to Iona Teeguarden, *The Acupressure Way of Health.*

The Eight Regulatory Meridians are grouped into the following four pairs:
- The Great Regulator ("Yin and Yang Wei Mo")*
- The Great Central Channel ("Tu Mo and Jen Mo"), commonly referred to as the Governing and Conception Vessels
- The Great Bridge Channel ("Yin and Yang Chiao Mo")
- The Penetrating and Belt Channels ("Ch'ang Mo and Tai Mo")

The Great Regulator is responsible for balancing all the functions of the body. It also controls the resistance to colds and flu by harmonizing the relation between the yin and yang organ meridians. Since the meridians influence our emotional states, the Great Regulator has been traditionally associated with pains in the heart, nervousness, timidity, fear, apprehension, mental depression, and nightmares.[16]

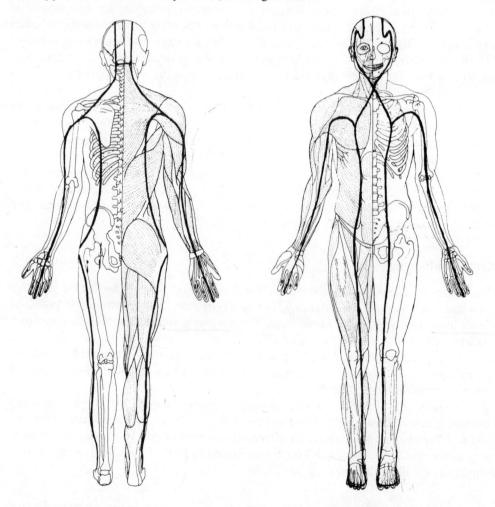

---

* "Yin" refers to the portion of the channel that flows along the front of the body, and "Yang" refers to the portion on the back.
[16] Felix Mann, *The Meridians of Acupuncture*, pages 117–118.

The Great Regulator Channel ("Yin and Yang Wei Mo") flows from both sides of the forehead to the temples, through the jaws, and the two sides then join at the throat. At the collar-bone, it again splits into two branches, and goes out over the chest. It then descends through the nipples, ribs, abdomen, groin, and travels down the insides of the legs to the ankles. The Channel goes through the toes to the outside of the foot, and ascends the outsides of the legs. The flow proceeds to the hips, up the sides of the back, across to the arms, and goes down the outer arms and through the tip of the third fingers. It then moves up the insides of the arms to the chest where it joins with the main branch. Another branch of the Channel goes from the outside of the upper arm up through the shoulders, neck, up over the head, to the forehead again.

The Great Central Channel is the only Regulatory Vessel that flows continuously through the body. (All the other Regulatory Channels flow only when necessary to balance the organ meridians.) As the most primordial vessel, the Great Central Channel is used in many Taoist meditations for unifying the mind and body. This channel benefits the central nervous system, strengthens the spine, and helps to harmonize spiritual unrest.

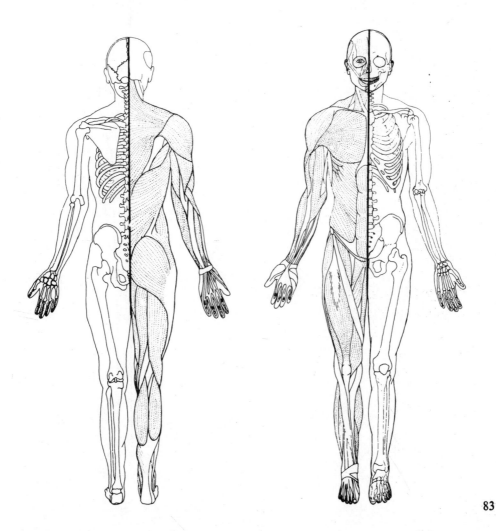

The Great Central Channel flows through the median line of the body. It consists of two parts: (1) the Governing Vessel, which travels from the perineum (between the genitals and the anus), up the spinal column, and over the head to the center of the upper lip; and (2) the Conception Vessel, which descends from the palate to the throat, and through the sternum, abdomen, and pubic bone to the perineum.

The Great Bridge Channel ("Yin and Yang Chiao Mo") functions to distribute the body's energy reserves. This energy ("Ching Chi") is stored in the kidneys, which are located in the lower back. The traditional Chinese doctors linked the body's energy reserves with the kidneys and the lower back as well as with the reproductive system. Basically, the Great Bridge Channel circulates to balance the deficient, weak areas (yin) with the excessively constricted areas (yang). This Channel is traditionally associated with aggressiveness, hypertension, fatigue, and lower back problems.

From the forehead above the eyes, the Channel goes down past the inside of the eyes and along the nose. It descends the face, and then travels through the sides of the throat,

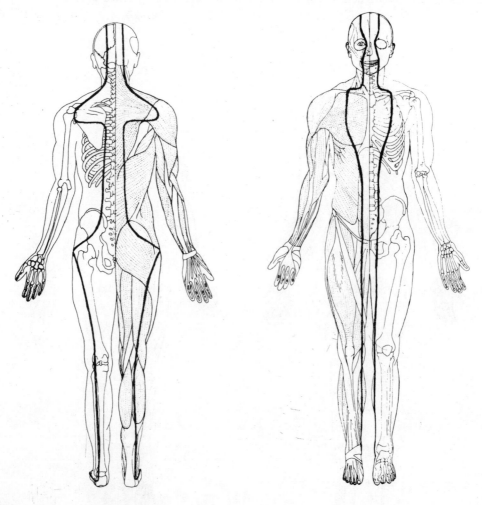

the chest, ribs, and abdomen. From the outer edge of the pubic bone, the Great Bridge Channel flows down the insides of the legs to the ankles, underneath the feet, to the outside corner of the little toe, and then up the outer sides of the feet. The flow penetrates up the outer back of the legs, takes a jog out toward the sides of the hips, then moves back over the buttocks, and ascends the back. At the middle of the shoulder blades, the Channel turns outwards toward the bottom of the shoulder, and then goes up to the tip of the shoulder. It proceeds up over the shoulders, up the back of the neck, and over the head to the forehead.

The Penetrating Channel ("Ch'ang Mo") circulates to balance all of the body's vital centers, the chakras. It is responsible for storing what the Chinese call "essential" energy. This energy is stored in the kidneys and linked with the genitals. At the time of orgasm, many times there is a warm penetrating feeling that travels up the front of the body from the genitals to the mouth.

The Penetrating Channel originates in the lumbar region, the lower back. It travels

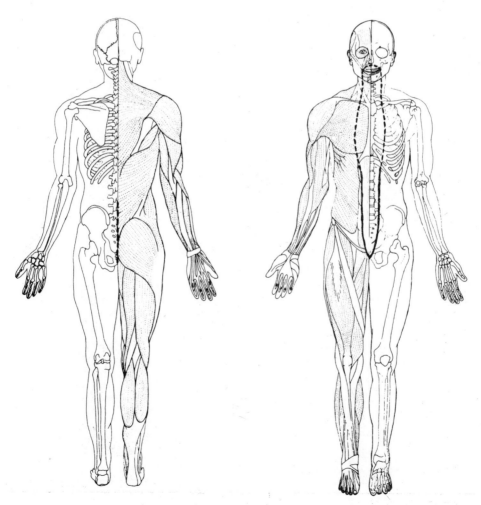

internally through the reproductive organs and penetrates up the front of the body near the midline, to above the upper lip.

The Belt Channel ("Tai Mo") circulates horizontally around the waist, dropping down to move across the abdomen at a lower level than across the back. It interconnects the organs in the abdominal area, and therefore is an important influence on the digestion. The Belt Channel is responsible for regulating our "gut level" feelings.

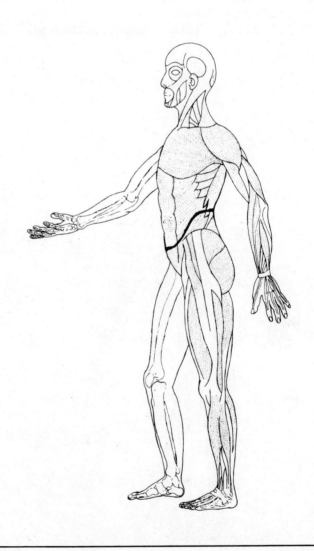

The Eight Regulatory Channels of Acu-Yoga
A Series of Exercises

Great Central Channel

Prayer Pose

A centering meditation based on the Great Central Channel.

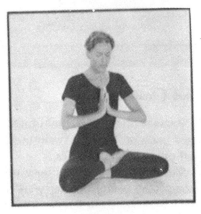

1. In a comfortable sitting position, place your palms together against the center of your chest, using the knuckles of the thumbs to press firmly against the point on the sternum at the level of your heart. This point (Conception Vessel 17) is the reunion point of all the yin meridians.
2. Close your eyes, straighten your spine, and breathe deeply into this point. This not only calms the nervous system, but opens up what the Chinese have called a "sea of energy" in the respiratory system.
3. Breathe long and deep, feeling yourself receive energy as you inhale. Allow this energy to circulate through your mind and body as you exhale. Meditate on the depth of your breath for one minute.

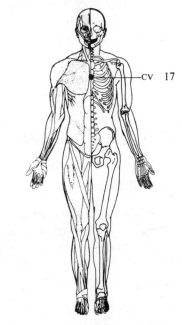

CV 17

Great Regulator

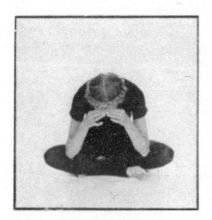

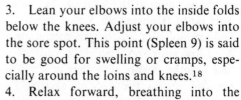

Mind Cleaning Pose

1. Remain sitting in a comfortable cross legged position. You may want to sit on a small pillow in this exercise.
2. Slowly lower your head forward, supporting it by gently placing your fingers on the forehead (Gall Bladder 14). A light touch on the forehead strengthens the emotional centers of the brain.[17] Use your thumbs to press on the jaw muscles (Stomach 6).

3. Lean your elbows into the inside folds below the knees. Adjust your elbows into the sore spot. This point (Spleen 9) is said to be good for swelling or cramps, especially around the loins and knees.[18]
4. Relax forward, breathing into the *Hara* (abdomen) for about one minute.

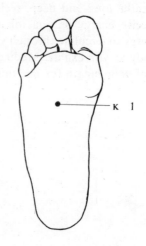

Great Bridge Channel

Extended Pose

1. Remain in a sitting position on the floor. Bend your left leg, and grasp hold of the bottom of the foot with your fingers. The point being stimulated on the sole of the foot (Kidney 1) is a strong phys-

---

[17] John F. Thie, *Touch for Health*, page 32.
[18] Felix Mann, *The Treatment of Disease by Acupuncture*, page 20.

ical revival point called "Bubbling Spring."

2.   Inhale and stretch this leg out in front of you at a 45 degree angle from the ground. Exhale and bring the leg down.

3.   After a minute switch legs and equally stretch the right leg. Work on the tighter side a little bit longer to help stretch it out.

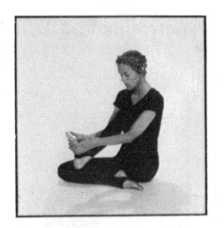

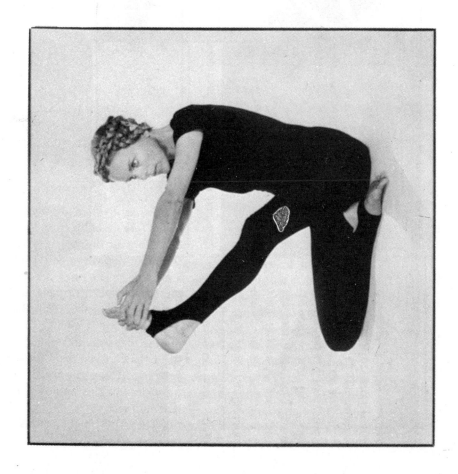

Penetrating and Belt Channels

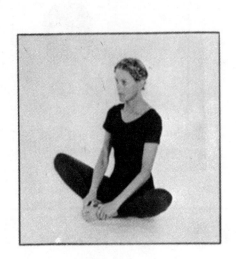

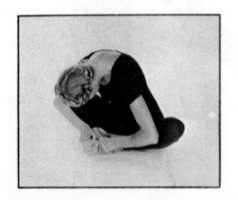

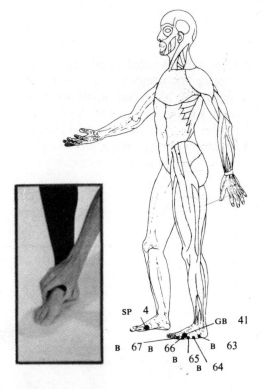

SP 4

GB 41

B 67 B 66 B 63

B 65

B 64

Butterfly Pose

1. Sit on the floor, bringing the bottoms of the feet together close to your genitals.
2. Use your thumbs to hold the point on the arches of your feet (Spleen 4). Use your fingers to press the point between the fourth and fifth metatarsal bones on the tops of your feet (Gall Bladder 41).
3. Inhale and straighten the spine, bringing the chest up and out.
4. Exhale as you bend forward, bringing your head forward towards your big toes.
5. Continue this up-down movement for one minute.
6. Then sit straight in this posture and breathe deeply.

Great Regulator

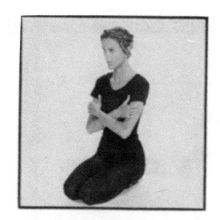

Cross My Heart Pose

1. Sit on your heels.
2. Cross your arms at your heart's center, holding the outsides of your upper arms. Use your third fingers to hold Large Intestine 14, just underneath the deltoid muscle on the side of the arm.
3. Inhale and straighten your spine.
4. Exhale, relaxing forward, forehead towards the ground, compressing the breath out. This position naturally puts pressure on several points including the master points of the Great Regulator (Triple Warmer 5 and Pericardium 6) which are located a couple of inchs above the wrists.
5. Stay down in this position a minute, visualizing a circulation of energy flowing up the back and down the front as you breathe. Then slowly return to an upright position.

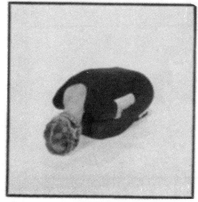

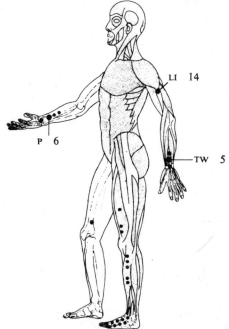

Great Central Channel

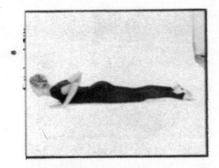

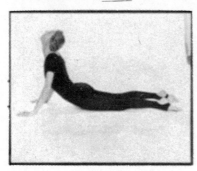

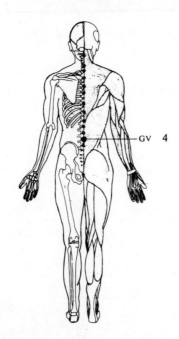

GV 4

Cobra Pose

1. Lie on your stomach with your chin on the ground. Bring your hands underneath your shoulders with the palms facing down.

2. Inhale and raise your head all the way up and back. Continue upwards, raising the upper portion of your body, keeping your pelvis on the ground.

3. Begin breathing into your *Hara*. The pelvic area is on the ground, the head is back, and the arms are straight, supporting some of the weight of the thoracic region.

4. After a minute or two in this position, exhale completely and squeeze your buttocks muscles, stretch back, and press your navel towards the ground. This will put even more pressure on Governing Vessel 4, the "Gate of Life."

5. Inhale deeply once again. Exhale and slowly come down by bending your arms. Feel a pressure in each vertebra progressively up from the lower to the middle parts of the spine as you descend. The head is the last part to come down.

6. Bring your hands to your sides, and let your head rest on its side. Relax and feel your blood circulate throughout your body.

All Regulatory Channels

Bow Pose

1. Lying on the floor on your stomach, bend your knees and bring your feet towards your buttocks. Rest your forehead on the ground.

2. Inhale and grab hold of the tops of your feet from the sides. Bring your fingers over the arches to hold Spleen 4 while the heels of your palms fit in between the bones on the outside of the tops of the feet.

3. Arch yourself back like a bow. Begin rocking as you inhale back and exhale coming forward. Breathe through your nose. Continue rocking back and forth for 15 seconds.

4. Come out of the pose slowly and lie flat. Relax for three minutes with your hands by your sides. Consciously breathe through your nose into and out of the *Hara*, the lower abdomen, during this three minute relaxation period.

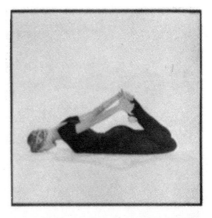

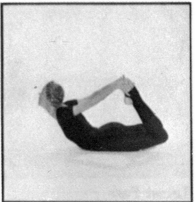

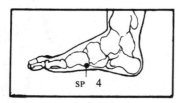

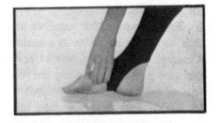

All Eight Regulatory Channels

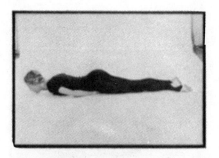

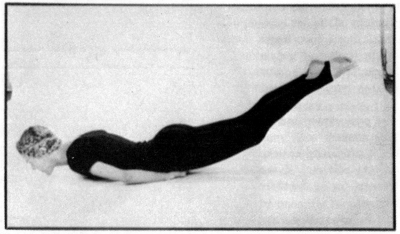

Locust Pose

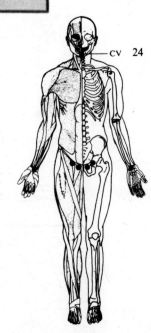

— cv 24

1. Lie down on your belly with your hands by your sides. Make firsts with your hands, and place your arms underneath your body with your fists on both sides of the groin area.

2. Bring your ankles together and your chin on the floor. There is a central point (Conception Vessel 24) below the lower lip that gets pressed by resting the front portion of the chin on the ground.

3. Inhale and raise the legs up. Begin *Hara* breathing with the legs held up for 30 to 60 seconds.

4. Allow your legs to come down and totally relax with your arms resting at your sides.

Great Regulator

Plow Pose

This pose also massages the internal organs, stretches the muscles along the spine, and helps to balance the thyroid gland.

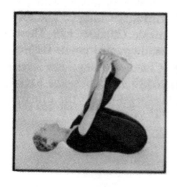 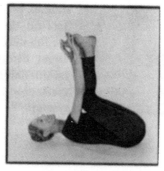 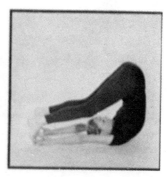

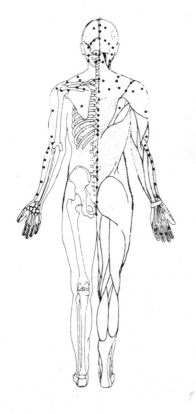

1. Lie on your back with your ankles together and hands at your sides.
2. Inhale deeply and raise your legs up to the sky.
3. Exhale as they come over your head towards the floor in back of you.
4. Bend your knees in this position, and bring your arms (also up and back) to your feet. Interlace your fingers inbetween your toes. This stimulates the Great Regulator which goes through the toes, the shoulders, neck and throat.
5. Practice deep breathing for about 30 seconds in this pose.
6. Slowly come out of the pose feeling a pressure on each vertebra as your legs come back to the floor. Immediately follow this pose with the next exercise to stretch the spine in the opposite direction, to avoid a buildup of pressure in the spine.

Great Bridge Channel

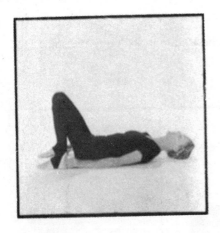

Under the Bridge Pose

1. Turn over on to your back. Bend your knees, bringing the bottoms of your feet on the ground near the buttocks.
2. Grasp hold of your ankles with your thumbs on the inside (Kidney 3) and fingers on the outside (Bladder 62). These are the master and coupled points for the Great Bridge Channel. They have been traditionally used to strengthen the back, the reproductive organs, and the urinary system.[19]

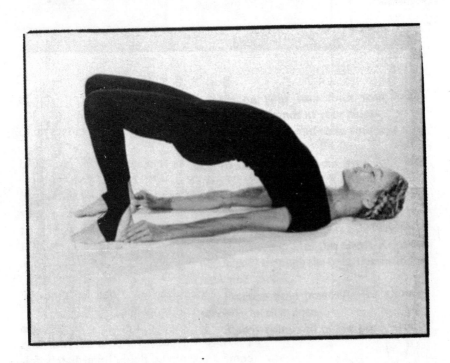

---

[19] Felix Mann, *The Treatment of Disease by Acupuncture*, pages 42, 44, 45.

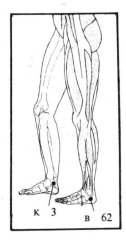

3. Inhale and arch the pelvis all the way up towards the sky. Hold this pose for 30 seconds. Breathe long and deep into the pressure being placed on the shoulders.
4. Relax down and lie quietly for a couple of minutes with your eyes closed. Visualize a current flowing through you.

Deep Relaxation

This reinforces all of the benefits of these poses and points. Let yourself completely relax on your back for about 10 minutes.

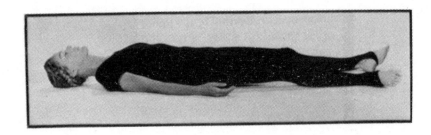

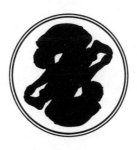

Chapter 6

The Organ Meridians

The organ meridians are distinct channels that circulate life energy, Ki, throughout the body. They are thought of as a master communications system of universal life energy, connecting the twelve organs with all other physiological, sensorial, and emotional aspects of the body. Over the past five thousand years, the Chinese have discovered hundreds of points that relate to the internal organs by way of the meridians. The twelve organ meridians are the Lungs, Large Intestines, Stomach, Spleen, Heart, Small Intestines, Bladder, Kidneys, Pericardium, Triple Warmer, Gall Bladder, and the Liver.

> *"It is said that in former times the ancient sages discoursed on the human body and that they enumerated each of the viscera and each of the bowels. They talked about the origin of blood vessels and about the vascular system, and said that where the blood vessels and arteries meet there are six junctions. Following the course of each of the arteries there are the vital points . . . . Each of these points has a place and name . . . and all have sections (meridians) which set them apart from each other."*[20]

The Chinese consider the meridians to be the web of life. They discovered that vital energy circulates through these channels, nourishing all systems of the body. According to the ancient Chinese teachings, these "rivers of health" flow continuously through the body.

There is a peak of energy which shifts from one meridian to another throughout the day, so that every twenty-four hours the Ki completes one cycle throughout the body. This crest of energy travels through each of the meridians at particular times according to the position of the sun. This creates a daily rhythm inside the body. There are times of the day when certain symptoms or feelings continue to reoccur. Everybody's daily pattern is dif-

---

[20] Ilza Veith, *The Yellow Emperor's Classic of Internal Medicine*, pages 117–118.

ferent. Some people awaken in the morning feeling groggy or irritable. This is when the Stomach and Spleen Meridians are functioning at their peak. Acu-Yoga poses that stretch or press points on these meridians could eventually help such a person.

The body clock illustrates a relationship between the meridians, the parts of the body where these meridians flow, and the times when this meridian is most active. For instance, many people commonly feel low or depressed in the late afternoon. According to Western physiology, fatigue at this time of day is partly caused by lower levels of blood sugar. This makes sense since we probably have not had dinner by this time. An Acu-Yoga perspective recognizes this physiological occurrence, but also realizes that the Bladder Meridian, which rules the back, flows most strongly between 3 and 5 P.M. Chronic back tension is as common as "the three to five blues." A great deal of muscular tension along this meridian may depress or block the natural flows at this time. According to the Chinese body clock, there is

The Body Clock

Legend (from the inside to the outside)
1. Time of day / 2. Name of the Meridian / 3. Brief rout description / 4. Association: sense, fluid, part of the body, taste / 5. Season, Climate, Emotion, Color

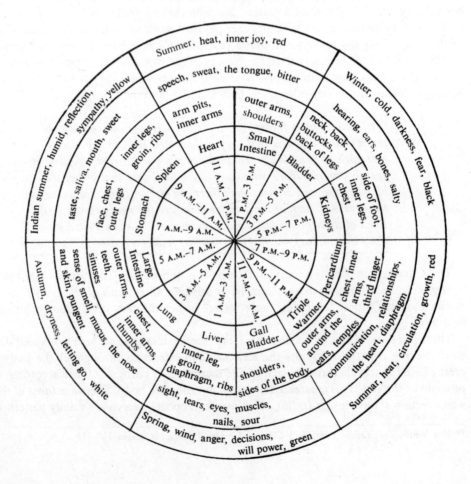

a relationship between the Bladder Meridian, the back, and the fatigue experienced at this time in the afternoon. So, only correcting one's blood sugar level may not be enough to counterbalance this kind of fatigue; releasing back tension may also be necessary. Many other relationships can be drawn to understand how to improve your individual condition through studying the body clock, the meridian associations, and the related Acu-Yoga exercises.

Acu-Yoga is based on these kinds of traditional Chinese teachings of holistic health. It works to release blockages and balance the essential life energy in the twelve organ meridians since each Acu-Yoga position works directly on meridian blockages. According to the Chinese, disease is the result of blockage of Ki energy in the meridians. This chapter covers exercises that activate each of the twelve organ meridians in the order of their flow.

Lung Meridian

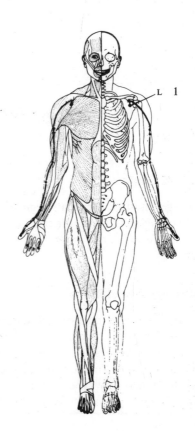

Meridian Route

The Lung Meridian begins at the outer portions of the chest, underneath the pectoralis muscles. From this point the Meridian travels along the insides of the arms, ending at the outside bases of the thumbnails.

Traditional Associations

The lungs control the body's physical energy through the depth of respiration or breath, which determines the amount of oxygen and Ki absorbed from the air. The Meridian also regulates the pores of the skin to adjust to variations in temperature and activity. Traditionally, the Lung Meridian is thought to protect the body from colds and flus. Strengthening this Meridian also helps to increase resistance to illness in general.

Lung Meridian Balancing Exercise

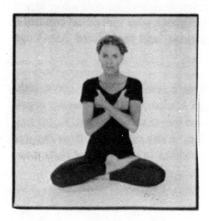

1. In a comfortable sitting position, interlace your hands at the center of the chest stretching your thumbs out so that they press into the muscles on the outside portion of the chest. This connects the beginning and ending of the Lung Meridian.

2. Close your eyes and begin long, deep breathing. Breathe into your abdomen first, allowing the diaphragm to open. The ribs then expand, and lastly the chest swells up to complete the full inhalation.

3. Hold the breath at the top of the inhalation for a few seconds. Then exhale, slowly releasing the breath gently and evenly. Continue for one minute.

4. Imagine a circuit of electricity or energy circulating through your mind and body as you allow your breath to be full and deep. This is only a breathing exercise, but it takes concentration and discipline.

Large Intestine Meridian

Meridian Route

The Large Intestine Meridian begins at the base of the index finger. It travels along the outside of the arms, where the two sides cross over the spine at the base of the neck. It then goes over the shoulders, around the neck, up the throat and over the jaws to a point beside the nostrils.

Traditional Associations

The Large Intestine functions to remove the water from and then eliminate solid wastes. It is responsible for cleansing, or detoxifying, on many levels. Physically it eliminates waste from the bowels; mentally it controls negativity and toxic thoughts, or what might be considered to be "mental constipation," and emotionally and spiritually it governs the ability to let go. Any type of constipation or holding is related to the Large Intestine, whether it is in a personal relationship, or with a possession, a thought, or an idea.

Large Intestine Meridian Balancing Exercise

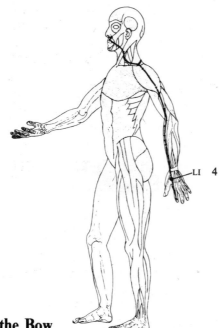

LI 4

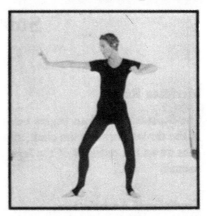

Opening the Bow

1. In a standing position, bring your arms up in front of you so that they cross at the wrists with your palms towards you.

2. Inhale and extend your right arm straight out to the side, bringing back the bow with your left arm. Face right, and point the index finger up with the nail facing you. This stretches the beginning of the Large Intestine Meridian.

3. Exhale as you release the bow, bending your arms so that the wrists cross in front again.

4. Repeat, this time to the left.

5. Continue this exercise, alternating sides, for one minute.

"Hoku" (Large Intestine 4), one of the most famous Acupressure points, helps to balance the colon. Its benefits are obvious from its name, "The Great Eliminator." It is traditionally used for constipation, frontal headaches, sinus problems, insomnia, nervous depression, stomach pains, and toothaches. The following Acu-Yoga posture stimulates Large Intestine 4.

Great Eliminator*

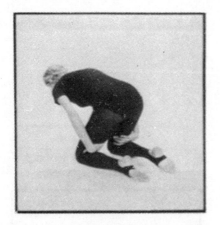 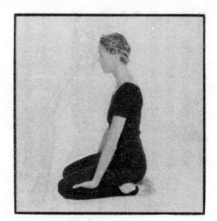

1. Sit on your heels in a kneeling posture.
2. Rock forward, and with the palms facing up, spread the index fingers and thumbs apart underneath your knees.
3. Lower yourself down, stretching the webbing between the thumbs and index fingers apart to press Hoku.
4. Stimulate the point by rocking back and forth as if you are on a rocking horse.

Stomach Meridian

Meridian Route

The Stomach Meridian begins below the center of the eyes. It descends down the sides of the throat, through the chest, nipples, abdomen, and groin, where it jogs over to and goes down the outsides of the legs, and over the instep, ending at the base of the second toenail.

Traditional Associations

Referred to as "the sea of nourishment," the Stomach controls the digestion of food. According to traditional Oriental health care, the Stomach is thought to be the most central organ of the body. Therefore, an imbalance in the Stomach will directly affect all the other organs.

---

* Since this exercise can trigger uterine contractions, pregnant women should not practice it.

Stomach Meridian Balancing Exercise

1. Kneel and sit on your heels. Take a deep breath with your spine straight.

2. Exhale, slowly lowering your chest to your knees, as your body compresses the breath out. In this position the movement of the breath internally massages the digestive organs.

3. Use your thumbs to press Stomach 3 (two fingers' width directly below your eyes), while you exhale coming down. Feel for a soreness or sensation at the point, pressing up against the cheekbone.

4. Repeat the first three steps for one minute, inhaling up and exhaling down.

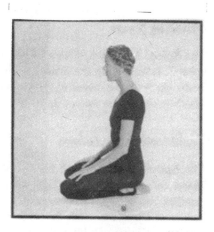

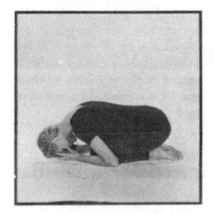

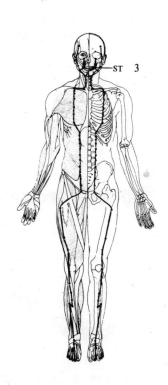

ST 3

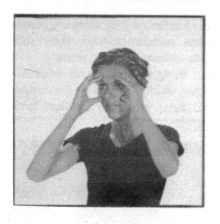

Spleen Meridian

Meridian Route

The Spleen Meridian, which includes the pancreas, begins at the inside base of the large toenail. It travels up the insides of the legs to the groin where it goes to the midline of the body, through the digestive organs, up over the ribs, and up to the outer part of the chest. The Meridian then moves down to end on the sides of the ribs, underneath the armpits.

Traditional Associations

The Spleen is responsible for storing blood, forming antibodies, and producing white blood cells which help to fight off poisonous bacteria. The classics say that the Spleen "unifies the blood." Consequently, menstruation is traditionally related to the Spleen-Pancreas Meridian. The Pancreas secretes enzymes that break down food into usable nutrients. It also regulates the blood sugar level through the secretion of insulin.

According to the Chinese teachings, the Spleen transports the energy in food up to the lungs. Here prana, the energy in the breath, combines with it to form the essential human energy that nourishes the whole body. In this way the Spleen serves an important role for developing human energy. If the Spleen-Pancreas Meridian is damaged due to worry, an excessive intake of sweets, or obsession, this process of food transformation will be hindered. In this condition a person may be weak, forgetful, worried, or have digestive problems.

Spleen Meridian Balancing Exercise

Locust Pose

1. Lie flat on your stomach, placing your arms underneath your body with your fists underneath your groin.
2. Bring your forehead or chin on the floor, whichever is most comfortable.
3. Bring your feet together. Inhale and

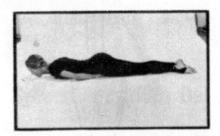

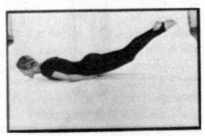

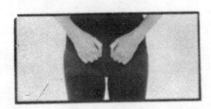

raise your feet up with the thighs off the ground. This puts pressure on many spleen and stomach points in the groin area where these two meridians tend to intermingle.

4. Begin long deep breathing with your legs up.

5. After 30 seconds, inhale deeply and stretch up. Hold the breath for 10 seconds.

6. Exhale coming down, and let go of your hands so that they relax at your sides. Adjust your body comfortably and completely relax.

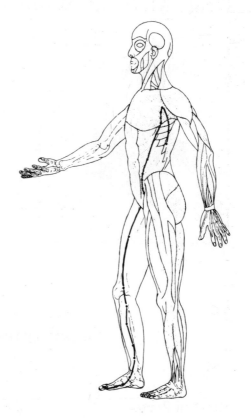

Heart Meridian

Meridian Route

The Heart Meridian begins in the center of the armpit and travels along the inside of the arm to the inside base of the little fingernail.

Traditional Associations

The Chinese classics say, "The heart is the root of life."[21] It is the seat of the spirit or *Shen*. As the ruling official or organ, the heart influences the overall stability of our emotions.

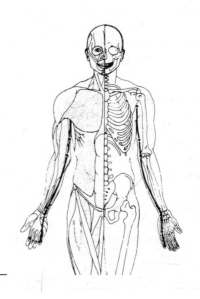

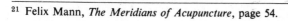

[21] Felix Mann, *The Meridians of Acupuncture*, page 54.

Heart Meridian Balancing Exercise

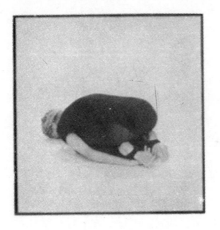

1. Sit on your heels. Bend forward, allowing your head to rest in front of your knees close to the floor.
2. Place your hands underneath your feet so that the palms are facing up. Take your little fingers and interlace them between your large and second toes.
3. Pretend you have a large tail and wag it. Continue moving your hips back and forth for one minute.

Small Intestine Meridian

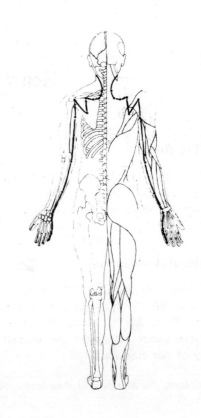

Meridian Route

From the base of the little finger, the Small Intestine Meridian runs along the outer arm to the shoulder, zigzags through the scapula, travels up over the shoulder, at the base of the neck, and ends in the face at the front of the ear.

Traditional Associations

The Small Intestine Meridian is responsible for the assimilation of the nutrients from food and the absorption of water. Mentally, the Small Intestine governs the assimilation of ideas. Elbow, shoulder pains, and stiff necks are common results of blockages of the Small Intestine Meridian, since it rules the shoulder blades and the joints.

Small Intestine Meridian Balancing Exercise

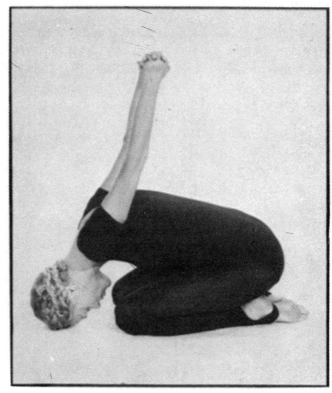

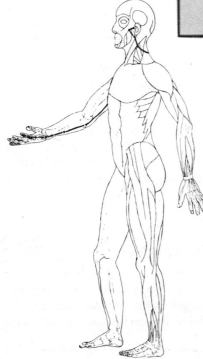

1. Remain sitting on your heels and lower your head to the floor. Interclasp your hands behind you, palms facing each other at the small of your back.

2. Inhale and stretch your arms up. Hold them up for 30 seconds, breathing deeply through the nose. This position will create pressures around the shoulder blades which releases tensions and is beneficial for building up resistance to colds and flus.

3. After 30 seconds inhale and stretch the arms up further. Then exhale and let the arms relax down by your sides, feeling the benefits.

Bladder Meridian

Meridian Route

The Bladder Meridian has more points than any other Meridian. It begins at the innermost corners of the eyes, and then travels over the skull, down each side of the spinal column, and through the backs of the legs, ending at the outside base of the little toenails.

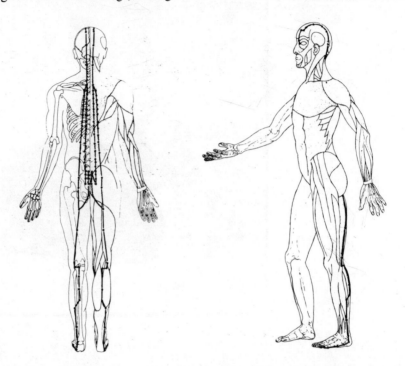

Traditional Associations

The Bladder Meridian is a very protective Meridian, accumulating a great deal of our physical and emotional tensions. It rules the back, the neck, the buttocks, the backs of the thighs, the calves, and the outside of the feet. It also has points which regulate all of the internal organs. Functionally, the Bladder is responsible for storing and excreting urine, which involves balancing the normal levels of fluid in the body.

Bladder Meridian Balancing Exercises*

Many people will find the Bladder Meridian stretch more difficult to do on one side than the other. This can be balanced by doing the exercise longer on the side that's tighter. Ease up a little when the stretch is painful and there is resistance. Remember that the fuller your breath is the easier the stretch will be.

1. Sit on the floor with your legs stretched out in front of you. Bend one knee, bringing your foot into the groin area, keeping the other leg stretched out in front of you.
2. Inhale and stretch up to the sky. Exhale and stretch down toward the extended leg keeping your shoulders relaxed. Pull your chin in slightly so your spine is in line. Exhale down, using your arm muscles to pull yourself further, bringing your forehead towards the knees.**
3. Continue for about one minute.
4. Before you switch to the other leg, stretch both legs in front of you and feel the difference. Close your eyes and wiggle your toes. Feel which one is lighter. If you look at your feet you might even be able to see a difference in coloration.
5. Switch sides, stretching out the other leg.
6. Finish by stretching both legs out in front again.

Now that you've stretched each leg individually, you're ready for the deeper stretch of doing both together, as in the following exercise.

1. Come to a sitting position with both legs stretched out in front of you. Rotate your feet and wrists a few times.
2. Grab hold of your ankles, or calves, wherever you can without straining and without bending your knees. Straighten

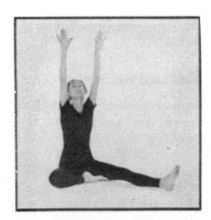

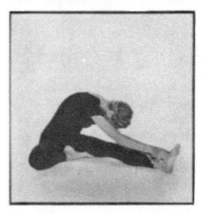

the spine and take a deep breath. The backs of the knees remain flat against the floor.
3. Inhale as you stretch up, and exhale bending forward, pulling yourself down with your arms.
4. Continue for one minute, establishing your own full breathing pace.

Kidney Meridian

Meridian Route

The Kidney Meridian begins at the soles of the feet, and travels up the innermost part of the leg, to the genital region. From the top of the pubic bone, the Meridian goes internally up to the tip of the coccyx, where it ascends the sacrum, lower lumbars, and goes into the Kidneys. An inner branch of the Kidney Meridian travels through the Kidneys, Liver, Heart, Lungs, and up the center of the throat into the ears. The main Meridian surfaces

* Variations of these exercises are referred to as Stretch Pose.
** Gently stretch into the position without straining.

above the pubic bone, flowing up the abdomen near the midline, to end just below the clavicle.

Traditional Associations

The Kidneys are traditionally considered the storage tanks of the body, gathering the surplus of energy and storing it to be used when needed. For this reason, the Kidneys are responsible for developing stamina. According to the Chinese, the Kidneys are also responsible for influencing sexual vitality. From the Kidneys reproductive energy is produced. Therefore an excess or lack of sexual desire is related to these organs. The Kidneys rule the bones, the ears, and our sense of hearing. Sensitivity to cold, ringing in the ears, semen leakage, and menstrual irregularity are some of the traditional associations of Kidney imbalances. If the Kidneys are strong, a person will have an abundance of vital energy.

Kidney Meridian Balancing Exercise

1. Sit on the floor, bending your knees and bringing the bottoms of your feet together. This pose joins both sides of the Kidney Meridian.
2. Hold your feet, using your thumbs to press Kidney 2 on both feet. This is an Acupressure point in the middle of the arch of the foot.
3. Pull your feet close to the genital area.
4. Inhale as you straighten your spine. Exhale and bend down, bringing your forehead down toward your toes.
5. Continue the movement breathing long and deep for one minute. This stretches the Kidney Meridian along the inner part of the leg.

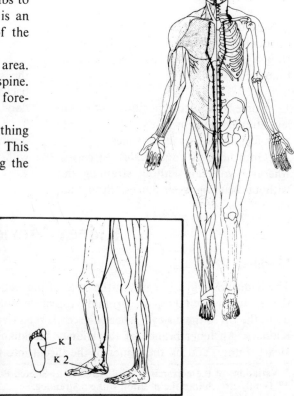

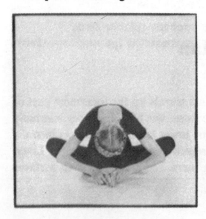

The Pericardium Meridian

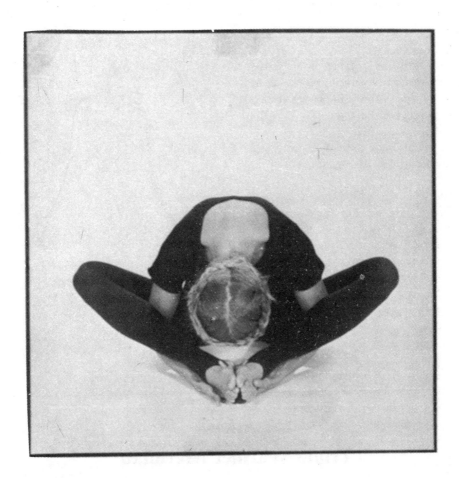

Meridian Route

The Pericardium Meridian begins in the chest muscles, just outside the nipple. It flows along the biceps muscle, through the inside of the elbow and the center of the inside of the arm, to the middle finger, ending at the tip of the middle finger.

Traditional Associations

Pericardium is sometimes called the "Heart Governor" or "Circulation/Sex" Meridian. It functions to protect the Heart, and is partially concerned with circulation. It also has sexual functions, as it connects with the Kidney Meridian. Emotionally, "the Pericardium is the organ from which the feeling of happiness comes."[22]

[22] Felix Mann, *Acupuncture*, page 83.

The Pericardium Meridian Balancing Exercise

1. Sit on the floor with the bottoms of your feet together.
2. Learn forward placing your wrists underneath your feet with the palms facing up. The outside of the ankle bones should be used to press Pericardium 7 (P 7), in the center of the wrist fold.
3. Allow your body to relax forward and breathe deeply in this position for 30 seconds.
4. Slide your hands two inches forward and apply pressure on Pericardium 6 (P 6), two inches above the wrist folds. Let your body relax forward for another 30 seconds.

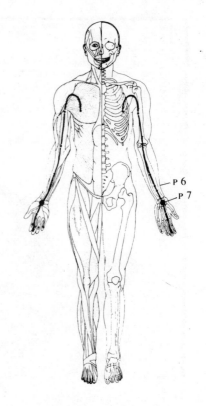

P 6

P 7

Triple Warmer Meridian

Meridian Route

The Triple Warmer begins at the ring finger. The Meridian travels along the arm, around the shoulders, up the outside of the neck, and around the ear to the temporal region.

Traditional Associations

There are three different sections in the trunk of the body. The upper segment, the "Upper Warmer," controls respiration, the "Middle Warmer" controls digestion, and the lower segment, the "Lower Warmer," controls elimination. In traditional Chinese health care, the Triple Warmer (the combination of these three) is considered a functional whole that helps to harmonize these three segments of the body. This Meridian also has the function of controlling body temperature and regulating the equilibrium.

Triple Warmer Meridian Balancing Exercise

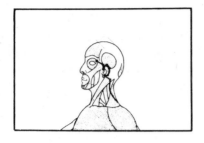

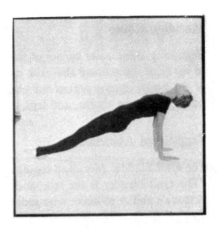

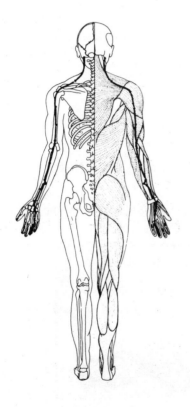

Platform Pose

1. Sit on the floor with your legs stretched straight out in front of you. Put your hands on the floor behind you with the fingers pointing away from your body. This should create a pressure in the hands and wrists, stimulating the Triple Warmer Meridian.

2. Arch the pelvis so that your body forms a straight line between knees and shoulders.

3. Begin long deep breathing or the breath of fire for one minute. You may begin to sweat. Impurities often come to the surface in this pose.

4. Relax on your back with your eyes closed, discovering the benefits.

Gall Bladder Meridian

Meridian Route

Beginning at the outer corner of the eyes, the Gall Bladder Meridian zigzags over the sides of the skull, goes down the back of the neck, crosses back over the shoulders to the front of the body, zigzags across the chest, and the sides of the trunk, then goes through the sides of the hips, thighs, and legs, ending at the second joint of the fourth toe.

Traditional Associations

The Gall Bladder Meridian regulates our ability to make decisions and to execute them. "The Gall Bladder is the true and upright official who excels in making decisions."[23] A persons's ability to make wise judgments is contingent upon the strength or weakness of the Gall Bladder Meridian. It also reflects our basic attitudes. If the Gall Bladder Meridian is too full, one easily can become angry or irritable. Indecision and muscular weakness would indicate a deficiency in this Meridian. It also controls the flexibility and strength of the tendons and ligaments. Migraine headaches that feel like a tight vise compressing the skull are a traditional Gall Bladder symptom.

Gall Bladder Meridian Balancing Exercise

1. Lie on your back, and then bend your knees to bring your feet up toward your buttocks.

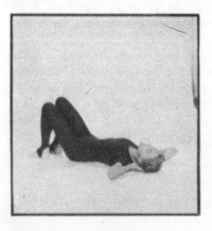 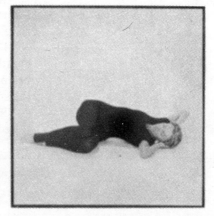

[23] Felix Mann, *Acupuncture*, page 95.

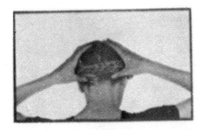

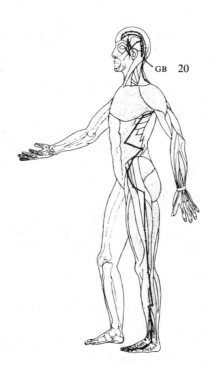

GB 20

2. Bring your hands underneath your neck. Press your thumbs underneath the base of your skull.
3. Inhale deeply. Exhale as you twist your body slowly moving your knees from side to side.
4. Continue for two minutes. Then relax flat on your back with your eyes closed.

Liver Meridian

Meridian Route

The Liver Meridian starts at the inside base of the large toe, travels up the inside of the leg and thigh, penetrates the male and female reproductive organs, and flows underneath the rib cage into the Liver, where it circulates internally up through the Lungs.

Traditional Associations

The Liver Meridian controls the eyes as well as the nervous system. The Liver secretes bile, which is necessary for the digestion of fats. Traditionally, allergies are related to the condition of the Liver. If this Meridian is too full, a person may easily get angry, whereas if there is not enough energy in the Meridian, a person is more likely to be depressed.

The Liver is responsible for planning in the way that the Gall Bladder controls our ability to make wise decisions and then carry them out. Together the Liver and Gall Bladder Meridians generate personal motivation and action.

Liver Meridian Balancing Exercise

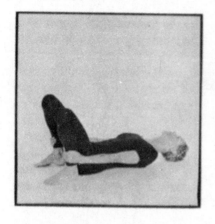 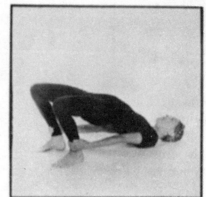

1. Lie on your back, bending your knees, and bringing your feet up towards your buttocks. Grab hold of your ankles, keeping your feet on the floor.
2. Inhale, arching the pelvis up, and exhale, bringing it back down.
3. After a minute, inhale and stretch up to the maximum. Tighten your buttocks muscles. Contract them, squeeze more, and relax the body down as you exhale.
4. Lie flat on your back with your eyes closed and relax completely.

Back to the Lung Meridian

1. Lie on your back and reach your hands for the sky.
2. Take a deep breath. Hold the breath in, make fists, and squeeze the muscles in your arms.

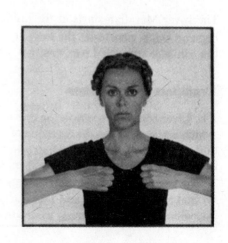

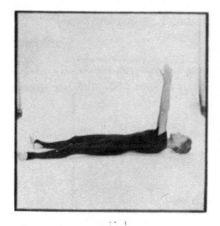 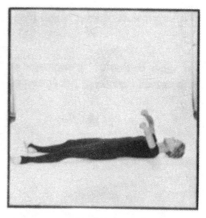

3. Slowly exhale, tightening the fists towards your chest. Continue four more times.

4. Relax on your back with your hands by your sides, palms facing up.

Final Deep Relaxation Exercise

Feel all parts of your body relax. Start with your toes and feet. Feel the legs, calves, behind the knees, buttocks and thighs relax. Feel all the organs in the abdominal area relax. Tell each vertebra from the base of the spine all the way up the back to relax. Relax the shoulders, the arms and relax each finger. Become very still. Tell the eyebrows, temples, and forehead to relax. Relax all across your skull, the ears and jaws. Feel your tongue, lips, and the roof of the mouth relax. Allow your eyes to relax. Let your mind relax, allowing your head to be clear. Enjoy the moment, letting yourself completely relax.

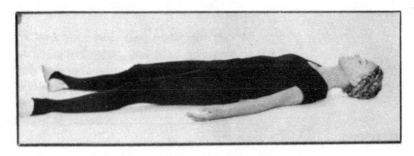

Third Deep Relaxation Exercise

Acu-Yoga Postures That Benefit Specific Conditions

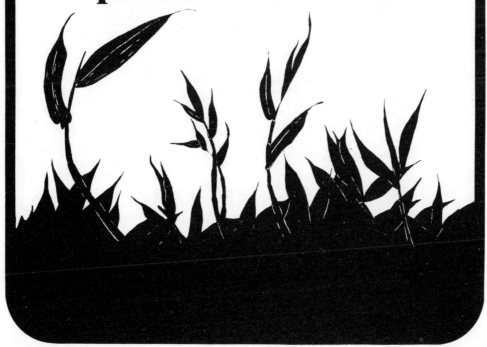

Acu-Yoga Postures That Benefit Specific Conditions

Although a holistic or whole-body approach is preferable, Acu-Yoga can also be practiced beneficially with a symptomatic orientation. This is because each pose stimulates specific points, meridians, and parts of the body traditionally associated with various conditions. These relationships are based upon centuries of observation and practice in the Far East. Although the symptomatic approach is limited it can be of value, often as a first step towards greater awareness of your body and its imbalances. Acu-Yoga enables you to do something for yourself, instead of always having to rely on others for information about your condition. The postures, breathing, and relaxation are a form of physical self-therapy that offers practical tools for enhancing one's health.

The symptoms we have are messages, or signals our bodies send us, indicating that there are more extensive, underlying imbalances that need to be attended to. Acu-Yoga does not treat symptoms or disease, or claim to cure health problems. In fact, many times the points and poses may bring a symptom to a peak, as buried or repressed problems begin to surface.

As we develop greater awareness of our condition, of our symptoms, and of our strengths and weaknesses, we also gain an opportunity to discover original causes of imbalance. The symptom is only a starting point, a key or clue to what needs attention. Through the practice of Acu-Yoga you may discover what you need to change in your life in order to solve the root of the problem.

Acu-Yoga thus attempts to prevent illness from occurring, rather than treating it. Acu-Yoga is a holistic method of health maintenance, not a form of medicine. If you have an illness or disease, please seek medical attention from a qualified doctor.

Although this section is organized symptomatically, it contains valuable information on many aspects of Acu-Yoga that apply to everyone, not just those with the particular symptom. Therefore, it's a good idea to read through all the sections, even the ones that don't seem to apply to you. You will probably find something useful anyway.

Each section includes a discussion of the topic, one or more Acu-Yoga exercises, and in some cases, other forms of self-treatment as well. The traditional associations are also included. A good method of practice is as follows:

Selection of Exercises

First of all, find several topics that relate to your condition, using the Table of Contents as a reference guide. Footnotes and cross references within a section will lead you to other topics. Explore the exercises which work on the areas you need. Select several of your favorites, including techniques that give you the most release during deep relaxation.

- Choose the four or five exercises that suit you best.
- Practice these exercises two or three times a day for one week, establishing Acu-Yoga as a daily routine. Gradually increase the length of time spent in each posture.
- Always follow your practice with 10 minutes of deep relaxation on your back with your eyes closed. Cover yourself with a blanket to keep warm and to enclose yourself, which helps you focus on the circulation of energy.

Through constant practice, Acu-Yoga can begin to improve your condition by releasing the tensions that cause or worsen it, and by balancing the body's Ki energy. This gradual but powerful process of regaining your health is referred to as Yogic therapy. As a highly developed form of holistic health care, Yogic therapy deals with all aspects of life, utilizing exercises, dietary principles, as well as postures, points, and breathing techniques. Acu-Yoga enables us to release the blocks that keep us from growing toward our own potential. Through it you can free yourself to experience the wealth of creativity, aliveness, and freedom that is your birthright.

Abdominal Weakness

Ideally, the abdomen is firm and also relaxed. It has good muscle tone without being rigid or hard, and is also flexible and soft without being loose or flabby. Few of us, however, are examples of the ideal!

Many people have weak abdomens, a problem which directly affects the intestines, the lower back, and the digestive and breathing functions. This is because over a period of time, weak abdominal muscles sag, and their digestive and eliminatory functions are weakened. This can be corrected by strengthening the abdomen.

The front and back of the body are directly related. Therefore, when the abdominal area is weak, the lower back is strained by having to compensate for that abdominal problem, which leads to weakening of the lower back as well. Many times lower back pain is accompanied by poor abdominal muscle tone, in which case it is just as important to strengthen the abdomen as it is to release the back tension.

Another consideration is that many of the abdominal muscles attach to the diaphragm, which expands and contracts with each breath. Therefore, tensions or flabbiness in the abdomen can also adversely affect breathing. With a strong and flexible belly, however, full and deep breathing is possible.

Healthy abdominal muscles are important for everyone, but are of special significance to women of child bearing age. If a woman decides to become pregnant the abdominal muscles must be strong to hold the extra weight of the growing child, and also to help the mother's body return to normal as quickly and healthfully as possible after the delivery. Poor muscle tone cannot accomplish this.

The Chinese connect the abdomen and the mind. If the abdomen is weak, then the mental facilities may be weak also; if the intestines are constipated, the thinking may also be clogged up. By strengthening our abdominal muscles and clearing the intestines with good diet and exercise, we can strengthen and clear the thinking also.

Proper muscle tone of the abdominal area is important for the proper alignment of the entire pelvic region. You can read the section on "Pelvic Tension" for another perspective on this.

Sit-ups are probably the best known exercise for strengthening the abdominal area. They are effective, but if you do them, be sure to bend your knees, because it prevents straining of the lower back by isolating the work of the exercise on the abdominal muscles alone.

But if you're bored with sit-ups, Solar Plexus Pose should do the trick! It strengthens the rectus abdominus muscles as well as the internal organs. You may have difficulty holding it very long, since it is a very rigorous exercise. Time yourself in the pose, and see if you can increase the length of time you can hold it by five seconds each time. Practice daily; build your muscles slowly. It's best to proceed slowly but surely.

Solar Plexus Pose also helps the body in another way: it activates the Solar Plexus, a large networks of nerves that join at the upper abdomen. Thus it helps strengthen the nervous system, so that it can channel more energy.

The nerves are replenished during sleep, when the body's metabolism slows down. Upon awakening, however, the body needs to adjust from the deep, unconscious state to the level of daily activity. Many people use coffee as a stimulant to help make the adjustment. But Solar Plexus Pose can awaken the metabolism more naturally by energizing the Solar Plexus, thyroid gland, and the nervous system.

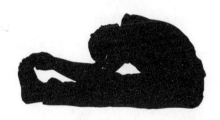

Solar Plexus Pose

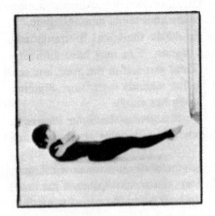

1. Lie on your back with your feet together.
2. Bring your arms around your chest, firmly hugging yourself.
3. Raise your head up and tuck your chin up into the hollow at the base of your neck.
4. Inhale, and raise your legs one foot off the ground, keeping your feet together.
5. Begin "Breath of Fire," rapidly pumping the air out your nose. (See p. 37 for a further description of this breath.) Continue for 20 seconds or until your body begins to shake.
6. Then completely relax with your eyes closed, allowing your blood and energy to circulate.

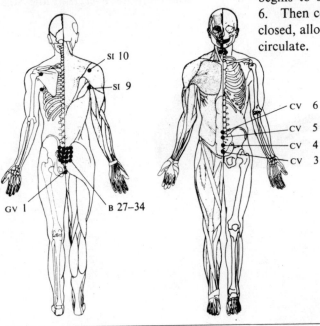

Acu Points	Traditional Associations
Small Intestine 9 and 10	Arm numbness or pain, arthritis, hypertension.
Governing Vessel 1 ("Long Stretch")	Nervousness, lower back and intestinal problems.
Stomach 9	Thyroid Gland.
Conception Vessel 3, 4, 5, 6 and Bladder 27–34	Abdominal weakness, bladder and reproductive organs.

Benefits: the arms, the nervous system, the Solar Plexus, colitis, thyroid irregularities, emotional imbalances.

Back Problems

Back problems are one of the most common ailments in our society. Almost everyone has experienced stiffness, tension, or pain in some part of their back, and some people suffer from it for years.

Back tension, stiffness, weakness, aches, and pains are a result of (1) lack of flexibility, (2) poor posture, (3) accidents, such as falls and car collisions, and (4) other stress, such as occupational or emotional pressures. These conditions affect the muscles and meridians of the back. The meridians become stagnated, blocked, or deviated, and muscular tightness builds up. Circulation is impeded as the toxic wastes of the metabolism cannot be properly carried away by the blood, so that the imbalance in the area is continued. Also, when one area of the back is stiff the body automatically compensates by taking pressure off that area and shifting it to another in order to relieve the strain and effort that can be caused even by common everyday movements. This, of course, shifts an extra burden of effort to another area of the back, compounding the problem.

Acu-Yoga, however, can release back tension and relieve pain. The stretching, strengthening and balancing techniques of Acu-Yoga have been used for thousands of years in the Orient to keep people well. Through the use of movements and postures that stretch the muscles and meridians and press certain points, Acu-Yoga effectively releases tensions and restores the natural harmony of the body.

Acu-Yoga also increases your awareness of your posture, of how you hold your body at all times and in all situations. As you cultivate this awareness, you can begin to work at correcting your poor postural habits. As your awareness grows, you will be aware of, and thus be able to correct any slumped-over or twisted positions you may find yourself in sooner than you otherwise would. This body awareness helps you to perceive an imbalance at an early stage of its development, so that you can do something about it before it grows into a larger problem. It's important to work on back pains as soon as you notice them, rather than "trying to ignore it" until it becomes so bad that the ache or pain becomes an unavoidable center of attention.

It is of utmost importance to keep your spine and your back muscles strong and flexible. The nerve segments of the back function as a network which directly affects all the organs and meridians of the body. This aspect of the nerves and spine is discussed in the section "Spinal Disorders."

The muscles of the back also have points which are directly related to all the internal organs and their functions. These are points on the Bladder Meridian which travels along the back muscles on either side of the spine. The points are known as Associated Points, or "Yu Points."

The Yu Points are located close to and on both sides of the spine, between the spine and the large sacro-spinalis muscles that run alongside it. The following diagram indicates the locations of the traditional Associated Points.

Thus, working to balance and strengthen the spine has a beneficial effect on all the organs. In general, the healthier the spine, the healthier the person is overall. This is why there is so much emphasis on the spine and back in Acu-Yoga.*

---

* Please see "The Flexibility of the Spine" under the chapter on the Basic Principles of Acu-Yoga.

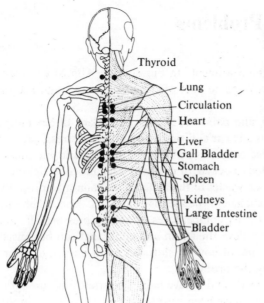

Thyroid
Lung
Circulation
Heart
Liver
Gall Bladder
Stomach
Spleen
Kidneys
Large Intestine
Bladder

Note that the points are generally located near the associated organ. Each specific area of the back relates to the internal organ that is nearby. Imbalances in the back can affect the organ, and problems in the organ can affect the back. In this way, back problems can express what is happening internally in the body.

Often back pains are the most severe in the morning, upon waking. The pain usually eases as the movement of daily activities stretches out the muscles a little. Heating pads or hot baths are helpful in that they can provide some temporary relief from pain and stiffness, but they do not usually change the condition more than that, unless used in conjunction with other therapeutics such as Acupressure or Acupuncture. Heat, in combination with regular practice of Acu-Yoga, deep relaxation, and meditation can give both short and long term results. Pressing the Acupressure points with warm towels can loosen the muscles up so that you can get more benefit from the postures. Deep relaxation and meditation after practicing Acu-Yoga balances and stabilizes the body's energies, providing a deep state of rest to counteract back tension.

Tensions in the **lower back** are associated with the Bladder, the Kidneys, and the reproductive system. Therefore, weakness of the Kidneys, which can be caused by eating too much salt, drinking too much liquid, an excess of sexual activity*, or from the emotion of fear, can cause problems in the lower back area.

Tensions in the **upper back** often have a psychological source. Curvatures, aches, or pressures in between the shoulder blades can be an expression of (1) the internal pressures created by pushing ourselves too hard, or (2) hurtful feelings lodged in back of the heart where the emotions of grief or loss are stored. In the first case, people who constantly drive themselves to do more than they can handle are constantly creating internal pressures and tension. What they do is never experienced as "enough." Consequently they have difficulty letting up the pressure on themselves. These inner pressures eventually cause knots of tension in the upper back, mostly between the shoulder blades and in the shoulders.

The second case is of people who do not allow themselves to experience the feeling of

---

* See "Potency" for discussion of the relationship between the kidneys and sexual activity.

loss or grief. Emotionally they tend to hold on to whatever has passed out of their lives. This difficulty in letting go automatically restricts the breath. Deep breathing can naturally release emotions. As emotional holding clamps down on the breathing and the emotional expression of the feeling, tensions around the chest and upper back result.

The Acupressure points in the upper back are related to the heart as well as to the lungs. For example, people with heart conditions or asthma almost always have tension in the upper back. By releasing the tension and balancing the energy, the heart and lungs benefit.

A word of caution: anyone with a back problem should be sure to practice Acu-Yoga carefully, to go slowly and gently in the postures. This is especially important for people who have long-term, chronic back problems, or people who have back injuries caused by an accident. No exercise should be practiced in a jolting or jarring fashion; no exercise should be pushed beyond your limit. STRETCH—DON'T STRAIN! If you are straining, you are doing it wrong! Do an exercise to the extent that it feels good, somewhere in between pain and pleasure. If a stretch "hurts good," then the level is right for you.

For example, say the pose is to bend forward, grab hold of your calf or ankle, and stretch your head towards your knees. This *does not mean* that to practice the pose "correctly," you should be in an extreme position, it means to gently stretch into the position as far as you can without straining. If the most you can do is drop your head and slightly round your shoulders forward, fine! Then that's your pose. Simply by doing that much you will gradually stretch out. ACU-YOGA IS NOT A CONTEST! Let go of your expectations and accept yourself the way you are.

Gradually, slowly, gently *ease into* the postures. Keeping your eyes closed allows you to get in touch with what you're doing, so that you can feel if you need to back off a little, go a little farther into it, or stay where you are for the moment. Get in touch with your own individual needs and limits. Appreciate what you *can* do, because if you accept your level and continue practicing, you automatically become more stretched out, more flexible. Accept, love, and appreciate where you are, and you will naturally improve the problems in the back.

The following two exercises, "Spinal Flex" and "Life Nerve Stretch," greatly increase the flexibility of the back. They both work on all the muscles of the back, benefitting the entire Bladder Meridian, and therefore all the internal organs as well (through the Associated Points).

The "Life Nerve Stretch" also works on the sciatic nerve that runs from the lower back down the backs of the legs. It stretches out the legs, hips, and back muscles, and is also good for urinary problems, cold feet, and stiff necks. "Life Nerve Stretch" is one of the most important and fundamental poses in Yoga.

Spinal Flex

1. Sit on the heels, placing the top (instep) of the left foot over the arch of the right foot.
2. Place the palms on the thighs, with the spine straight.

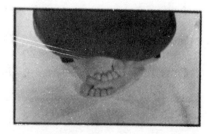

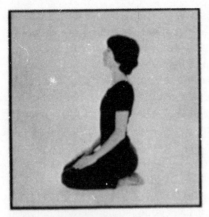
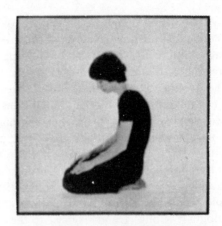

3. Inhale and flex your spine forward. Arch the spine gently but firmly in this forward motion.

4. Exhale and let the spine slump back. This stretches the spine in the opposite direction. Let your head simply rest on your neck, moving slightly with each flex of the back.

5. Continue for one minute. Begin slowly and gradually, feeling the motion and stretch in your back. Gradually increase the speed as your back loosens up. Breathe with each movement, inhaling as the chest pushes open and forward, and exhaling back and down.

6. Relax on your back for a few minutes.

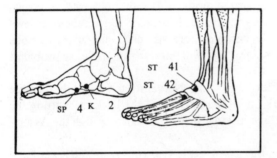

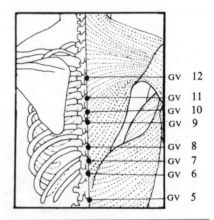

Acu Points	Traditional Associations
Spleen 4	A reflex point for the mid-upper back, digestive problems, abdominal pain, muscle cramps.
Kidney 2	A reflex point for the middle of the back, cold feet, chest or abdominal pain, swelling.
Stomach 41, 42	Often cold, walking around aimlessly, vertigo, madness, and fits.
Governing Vessel 5 through 12	Back stiff and painful, loins and spine rigid, nervousness.

Benefits: spinal stiffness, back aches and pains, indigestion, nervous disorders, postural problems.

Life Nerve Stretch

1. Sit with your legs together, stretched out straight in front of you. Keep your knees straight.

2. Exhale and lean forward. Depending on how stretched out you are you may hold your knees, calves, ankles, feet, or large toes.

3. Continue for one minute, inhaling up and exhaling down. Start very slowly, feeling the stretch and the rhythm of your breath. The deeper your breath, the easier it is to stretch the back and legs.

4. Lie back and relax for a few minutes. Be sure to follow this exercise with "Cobra Pose," (in *Spinal Disorders* section) to stretch the spine in the opposite direction.

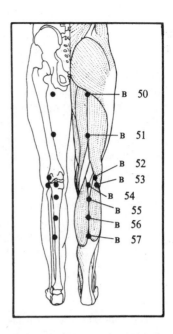

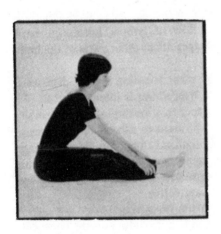

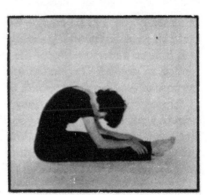

Acu Points	Traditional Associations
Bladder 50	Hemorrhoids, constipation, lumbago, sciatica, pain in the back.
Bladder 51	Inability to bend up and down easily, pain in the back and loins.
Bladder 52, 53	Muscular spasm of the calf, knee and loin pains.
Bladder 54, 55	Body feels stiff and heavy, stiff back and neck, arthritis of the knee.
Bladder 56, 57	Pain in calf and instep of foot, muscular cramps.

Benefits: sciatica, urinary and bladder problems, stiffness or pain behind the knee, muscular spasms, cold feet, late afternoon fatigue, leg stiffness or pain.

Body Tension

Every tension you have has a cause that lies behind it. Ask yourself, "What is causing me to be tense? What am I tensing against?" It could be many things: a relationship, work, anger or other feelings, fatigue, even how you feel about yourself or your attitude about life in general.

A good exercise is to focus on your tension. Read through this paragraph, and then take a few minutes to practice this simple body-awareness technique:

> *Close your eyes and put your attention on your body. "Look" for the tight areas; explore where you hold tension, and what is causing it. If your shoulders and neck are tight, ask them what has and is continuing to cause them to be that way. Keep your eyes closed and let your mind open up; a few simple words may come to you if you take the time to look clearly at what is there.**

Tension, where the muscle fibers remain in a tensed, contracted state, can be one of the preliminary stages of disease. It blocks the natural flow of lymph, hormones, nerve impulses, blood, and Ki energy. Eventually these blockages affect other parts of the body, creating weaknesses and lowering resistance.

A holistic understanding of the body is necessary whether releasing specific diseases or tension in general. Our bodies are one complete unit, everything is interconnected. The purpose of Acu-Yoga is to unite the mind and body into a relationship of deep harmony.

Tension can be a great learning tool. It guides us to the areas or aspects of ourselves we need to work on. You can use your tension as an individualized clue, or guide, for change. But if you block out what is making you tense, if you suppress or avoid your feelings, then the tension accumulates. Accepting yourself the way you are, here and now, going with your feelings and learning from them, is the highest way to live.

Many times tension is caused by excess. Amounts of food, exercise, work, and rest influence your physiological balance. The healthiest foods turn into poison when eaten excessively. Too much rest or activity also causes problems; the key is to discover your own personal needs for balance, and remember that quantity affects quality.

A Zen monk once learned a most enlightening meditation, and decided to practice it for the rest of his life. During the first two weeks heat, color, and light circulated throughout his body. But after a month of only sitting, his body became cold and weak, and even began to get sick, forcing him to change. A balance of activities and rest is necessary for maintaining health.

Food can also cause tension. Oriental peoples have studied the relationship between food and tension for centuries.** Certain foods cause extreme biochemical reactions. Salt, for example, has a binding effect on the tissues and organs: when put on a cut, salt will

---

* The "Meditation for Exploring the Cause of Disease" has a more expanded explanation of the process, and you may wish to refer to it now, page 44.
** Ohsawa, George, *Zen Macrobiotics*, Pocket Book Editon (Los Angeles, 1965).

cause it to close up. In excess, it is associated with high blood pressure and hardening of the arteries. Meat can also produce muscle tension. It contains salt, saturated fats, and uric acid, which contract the muscle fibers. If the uric acid is not eliminated through proper exercise, it accumulates and contributes to overall body tension.

This next exercise, "Boat Pose," presses on the solar plexus, and helps to release a central Acupressure point (CV 12) located between the navel and the breastbone. Long, deep breathing in this pose releases overall body tension. Try to practice this exercise for 30 seconds, relaxing immediately afterwards for a few minutes, with your eyes closed and your hands by your sides. The relaxation after this Acu-Yoga pose is vital for replacing your tension with a circulation of energy.

Boat Pose stimulates points on the Stomach and Kidney Meridians, as well as on the Conception Vessel. It's also beneficial for developing stamina, concentration, strengthening the lower back, improving circulation, and balancing the abdominal area.

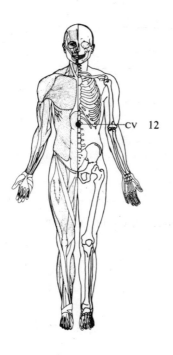

Boat Pose

1. Lie on your stomach, feet together and arms at your sides. Rest your head on your chin.
2. Stretch your arms so that they are straight in front of you, and on the floor.
3. As you slowly and deeply inhale, arch back, lifting your arms, chest, head, and legs off the ground.
4. Begin long deep breathing. Push beyond the time you think you can hold the pose, working up to 30 seconds.*
5. Completely relax for at least three minutes with your arms by your sides and your head turned to the side.

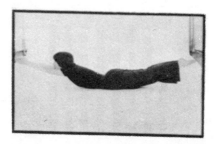

* People with high blood pressure should not push themselves with this pose. Those who have chronic heart conditions should not practice this exercise. People with acute or mild cases of hypertension may do this pose gently for five to ten seconds at a time. These people must allow themselves several minutes to completely relax after practicing the exercise to obtain the therapeutic benefits.

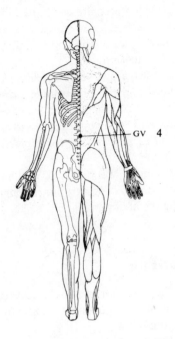

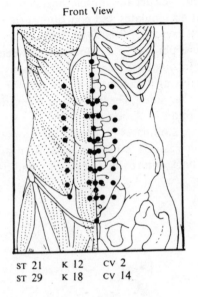

Front View

GV 4

| ST 21 | K 12 | CV 2 |
| ST 29 | K 18 | CV 14 |

Acu Points	Traditional Associations
Kidney 12–18 } Stomach 21–29 }	These points can release abdominal distension, aches and pains, digestive and intestinal problems.
Conception Vessel 2–14	Overall body tension, internal nourishment, and rejuvenation.
Governing Vessel 4	"The Gate of Life."

Benefits: kidneys and adrenal glands, abdominal distension, pain or cramps, overall body tension, lower back problems, fear, fatigue.

Circulation

Over four thousand years ago, *The Yellow Emperor's Classic of Internal Medicine* described the circulation of the blood, which was not discovered by Western physicians until the sixteenth century. Since ancient times, Acupressure and exercise techniques have been used in the Orient to improve circulation.

Physical Influences

A majority of circulation problems are caused by muscular tension and lack of exercise. Muscular tension blocks proper circulation because the contracted muscular tissue physically constricts the arteries and veins, and therefore constricts the flow of blood. The chronic muscular "armoring" can greatly imbalance areas of the body, blocking circulation.

Lack of exercise also contributes to poor circulation. Exercise stimulates the heart to pump faster and stronger, increasing the circulation to get the necessary oxygen to the cells of the body. Physical exercise moves the body, warms it up, stretches and loosens tendons, and releases tension in the muscles.

Poor circulation is a self-perpetuating negative condition. That is, if an area is imbalanced so that the circulatory flow is impeded, then the lack of circulation itself causes further imbalances. When the blood cannot properly get to the cells to bring oxygen and nutrients, and flush away waste materisls, then the cells and tissues become undernourished, and toxins accumulate, thus furthering the stagnation and tension in the area.

Acu-Yoga improves circulation in two ways. Firstly, by working directly on the Acupressure points, the tension in an area can be released. Secondly, as a highly developed form of physical exercise, Acu-Yoga stretches the muscles and moves all parts of the body. Through daily practice, the elasticity of the arteries can improve. The combination of Acupressure and Yoga effectively opens up the blood flow, so that fresh nutrients can circulate and toxins and other acidic wastes can be carried off for excretion.

Circulation problems are commonly caused by shoulder and neck tension in particular. Since poor circulation often manifests as cold hands or feet, Acu-Yoga exercises release points that can increase the blood flow in those areas. During the deep relaxation following the exercises, people often experience rivers of warmth flowing into their extremities.

When the weather is cold so that someone with poor circulation feels uncomfortably cold, her or his tendency, unfortunately, is to tighten up. Of course the exact opposite of that is what brings relief, namely, relaxing with the cold. When you tighten against cold, you simply create more tension and thus less circulation. So, the next time you're cold, take a big, deep breath and RELAX! Move your body, breathe, let go, and feel the circulation of the blood and energy. Fighting the cold doesn't work, flowing with it does!

Dietary Considerations

There are some dietary considerations related to circulation. If your body feels cold, especially your hands or feet, this is considered a yin condition—cold being an attribute of yinness. This yin condition may be caused by, or worsened by, eating too many yin foods.

To balance this, limit your intake of alcohol, fruit, honey, fluids, and cold or chilled foods. Especially be sure to eliminate foods that contain white sugar, which is extremely yin.*

Sautéed onion, ginger, and burdock root are three foods which help aid circulation. Miso soup** is excellent for general strengthening and effectively warming up the body. In general, of course, hot foods heat up the body, and cold ones cool it down. Some hot foods, however, such as "spicy hot" ones—chili, curries, etc.—do heat up the body, but are also irritants to the system when eaten in excess. Buckwheat is considered one of the most yang, heat-producing vegetarian foods. To achieve balance, in general, all foods should be eaten in moderation.

The following Acu-Yoga exercise, "Plow Pose," interlaces the hands and feet in a traditional Yogic position for reawakening blocked Ki. Immediately after practicing the pose lie flat on your back with your eyes closed, relax, and feel the increased circulation of the blood.

Plow Pose also regulates the internal organs and assists in weight loss. It improves the circulation by temporarily increasing the blood pressure. People with a high blood pressure condition*** should be careful not to push themselves in this posture. For example, start with 10 seconds, and only increase the time gradually. Relaxation afterwards is required.

Plow Pose

1. Lie on your back with your legs straight, your feet together, and your hands at your sides.
2. Inhale deeply, and as you exhale, raise your legs up and over your head bringing your feet toward the floor behind you. Keep your legs as straight as possible.

3. Reach back, grab hold of your toes, and interlace your fingers in between them.
4. Let your body relax. Breathe deeply. Concentrate on circulating your attention through your entire body, and visualize a current of energy flowing through you.
5. After 30 to 60 seconds, bring your arms to their original position on the floor. *Slowly* bring your legs back up and over so

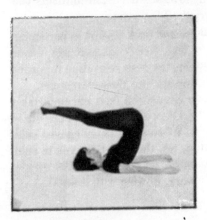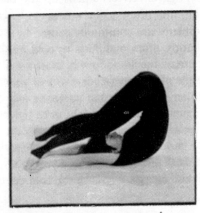

---

* If you have the opposite condition and are generally very warm, intense, and hyperactive, balance this yangness by avoiding extreme yang foods, such as meat and salt.
** *Miso* is a traditional Oriental food made from aged soybeans and salt. Consult a health food store for cookbooks with recipes for dishes using *miso*.
*** See section on "Hypertension."

that you are lying flat on the floor again. Keep your legs straight while you're bringing them down.

6. Completely relax for a few minutes on your back. Follow with Cobra Pose (under "Spinal Disorders," page 228), or Bow Pose (under "Indigestion," page 181) to stretch your spine in the opposite direction.

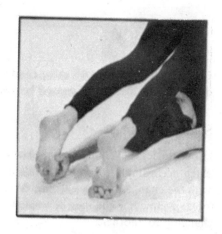

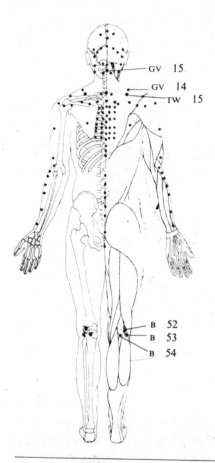

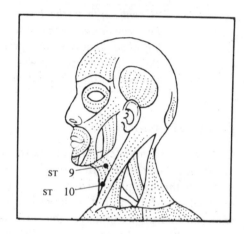

Acu Points	Traditional Associations
Bladder Meridian	The back, urination, and the sciatic nerve.
Extremity points	Improvement of circulation.
Bladder 52, 53, 54	Constipation, knee and abdominal problems.
Triple Warmer 15	Neck, shoulder, back painful or stiff.
Stomach 9, 10	Swollen or sore throat, thyroid problems.
Governing Vessel 14, 15	Headache, neck stiff, spine rigid.

Benefits: cold feet, shoulder tension, uptightness, fever, abdominal distension, fear.

Colds

Colds are associated with three conditions: change of the seasons, emotional holding, and diet. Each of these is discussed below.

Seasonal Changes

For centuries the Chinese have observed the changes of the weather and have dressed and eaten accordingly to prevent colds and flus. Colds indicate that we are out of harmony with the changes of the seasons. When a person's resistance* is low, one's ability to adapt to environmental changes is weakened, and it's easier to get a cold when one season is changing to another.

> *"Change affects the body and thus brings disease . . . .*
> *The troublesome winds affect [colds] beneath the lungs, bring-*
> *ing about illness in this place . . . .*
> *Saliva and mucus appear; evil winds then bring chills, and*
> *this causes the illness of the troublesome winds."*[24]

Emotional Considerations

Colds can be a manifestation of unexpressed emotions. Normally the body functions to maintain balance, but if your emotions are not expressed directly, they are often released indirectly through physical symptoms. Thus it is not at all unusual for a person to release or expel stressful emotions indirectly through the cleansing process of a cold. Repressed tears can change into mucus as they drip down internally from the tear ducts into the nose. Emotionally caused colds are generally an expression that the body needs to slow down or cleanse itself in order to regain balance.

Dietary Considerations

Colds can also be a process of cleansing excess mucus and toxins. A person who has eaten a significant percentage of devitalized foods (canned, processed, refined, preserved), white flour, white sugar, or salt accumulates toxins and mucus in the system. As you begin to drop these processed foods from your diet, however, your body naturally starts to cleanse itself. Thus, a person who begins eating a simpler, cleaner, healthy diet who gets colds is actually in the process of getting healthier. In this case a cold is *regenerative*, not *degenerative*. The cold, or cleansing, is actually a "healing crisis" where the body releases toxicity at a fast rate.

Once you begin to clear up your system, the knowledge of balancing your diet in terms of the yin and yang elements becomes important. This is a holistic way of balancing your diet. A knowledge of the yin and yang properties of foods and their effects on the body

---

* Please see the section "Resistance to Illness" for further discussion.
[24] Ilza Veith, *The Yellow Emperor's Classic of Internal Medicine*, Chapter 9; Section 33, page 138.

explains a lot of things about diet that often puzzle people. It is probably best illustrated by the story of my own personal experience with colds.

I used to catch one cold after another. Being absorbed in a variety of health practices, such as Yoga, meditation, and a natural food diet, I could not understand why I kept getting colds. Especially since I made sure I ate lots of oranges, which are high in Vitamin C. I was under some stress from school, sure, but why should a health-minded person like myself catch so many colds?

It seemed strange to me that my Acupressure teachers didn't mind giving me treatments or having me babysit while I had a cold. Why didn't they want to protect themselves from my germs? They didn't seem to get sick in the winter, or be bothered by the cold weather like other people I knew. What made them different?

While babysitting for them I got a clue. I would go through their refrigerator to check out what there was to eat. They certainly ate well—thick soups, homemade wholewheat bread, vegetables, brown rice—but there was hardly anything to munch on.

Weeks went by until I finally felt ready to receive a new idea. I now wanted to learn how to prevent colds and flus even if I had to change my life a little. I therefore approached one of my teachers for advice.

"The most important traditional principle of health," he said, "is to use moderation. The body expels excess to maintain balance. You are expelling mucus which is yin. Therefore, you are probably eating too many yin foods such as fruit (especially tropical fruit juices), ice cream, sweets, and so forth. You tend to eat in excess what you enjoy most, but even the healthiest foods are poisonous when eaten in excess. Remember to eat a *balance* of foods—be aware of the percentages between the yin and yang foods in your daily diet. Think of your favorite foods and count how much of them you eat in one day. Become aware of what you eat in excess and consciously eat less of those foods, to most effectively balance your condition."

Upon reflection I realized I was eating four to eight pieces of fruit a day. I thought, "But fruit is supposed to be good for you," and then realized that the issue of "good" or "bad" was not the question, as much as the issue of balance was. Even "good" foods become "bad" when eaten in excess. A healthy diet is one in which yin and yang are balanced, since *any* excess causes imbalances. Therefore I decided to limit myself to one piece of fruit a day.

Still, I did not believe this would prevent me from catching so many colds. I went back to my teacher to express my doubts, and to ask what foods I should eat in place of the fruit that I had been eating excessively.

"Sprouts, vegetables, and whole grains are considered the most balanced foods according to traditional Oriental health care," he replied. "It will take time for your body to readjust. You probably will still expel mucus, but not as much or as quickly. After a year of eating a balanced diet* you will not catch as many colds. In the meantime, learn how to adapt your diet to be in harmony with the changes of the seasons."[25]

---

* Balanced in regards to yin and yang.
[25] Please refer to *Healing Ourselves* by Noboru Muramoto for information on this topic.

I tried it . . . just as an experiment, though. But that was four years ago, and now I can say that it works! This kind of diet not only helps expel mucus and toxins, but it strengthens the body's resistance. Both aspects help prevent colds.

The Process of a Cold

During a cold the body goes through many internal changes. The Chinese observed that these changes vacillate between yin and yang. Yin symptoms change into yang symptoms and vice versa.

Colds often start when we are tired, or under stress. Our system is most receptive to catching a cold when our resistance is low. The body gets chilled in this yin (unprotected) condition. Yin (cold) changes to yang (heat) as our body generates heat to protect itself, resulting in a fever. Chills or sweating may follow to cool the body down. Sinus congestion or headaches, runny nose, chest congestion (from the mucus of the runny nose settling in to the lungs), coughing (to expel the mucus in the congested chest), sore throat (from all the coughing), and phlegm can follow.

Symptoms of a cold do not always evolve in this exact order, but the order of symptoms listed above does illustrate the dynamic process where a yin symptom becomes a yang one and vice versa. These changes are the body's attempt to regain internal balance.

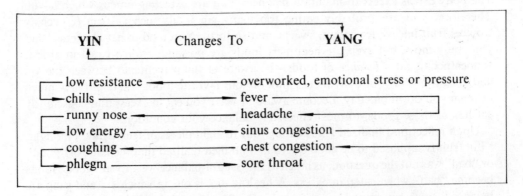

Remember that a cold is a cleansing of excess; if you aren't hungry, DON'T EAT! Let your digestive system rest, as well as resting in general, so that your body can use its energy to "clean house."

The Yellow Emperor asked his wisest minister, Ch'i Po, why colds and symptoms sometimes linger on. Ch'i Po answered:

"All these remnants of illness are caused when the patient was made to eat too much while the fever was high. All this means is that the illness has retreated but the heat [fever] is still within the body, because the energies of the foods attack each other and two elements of heat join together so that the fever remains . . . . When the illness of heat [fever] shows little improvement and the

patient eats meat, there will be a relapse; when the patient eats much there will be a remnant."[26]

The following Acu-Yoga exercise, "Half Wheel Pose," is good to practice gently when you have a cold; it can also help prevent colds by releasing blocked toxins and energies:

Half Wheel Pose*

1. Lie on your back. Bend your knees and bring the bottoms of your feet flat on the floor.
2. Loosely cup your hands, and then bring them under your neck with the knuckles together. The backs of your hands are together and your pinky finger knuckle presses into the base of the skull as shown.
3. Spread your index finger and thumb apart on each hand, creating pressure on Large Intestine 4 ("Hoku").
4. Inhale and arch your hips up. Breathe deeply into your *Hara*.
5. Continue breathing in this position for one minute.
6. Exhale and slowly come down. Cover yourself with a blanket and allow yourself to deeply relax on your back.

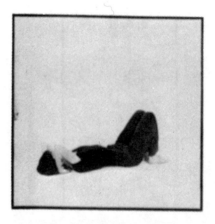

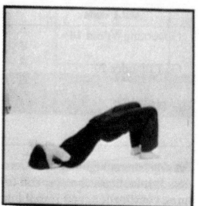

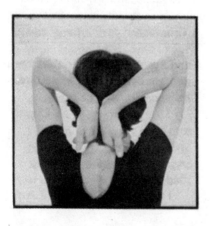

[26] Ilza Veith, *The Yellow Emperor's Classic of Internal Medicine*, Chapter 33, page 241.
* Do not practice this pose during pregnancy. Large Intestine 4 can cause the uterus to contract when it is stimulated strongly. This point is used during labor.

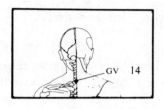

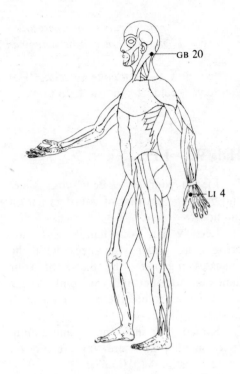

Acu Points	Traditional Associations
Governing Vessel 14	Colds, influenza, fever, vomiting, stiff neck, coughing, convulsions in children.
Gall Bladder 20	Headache, colds, influenza, fever, coughing, eye problems.
Large Intestine 4	Constipation, frontal headache, sinus trouble, colds, influenza, coughing, sore throat, menstrual difficulties.

Benefits: migraine headaches, menstrual tension, facial and eye disorders, shoulder tension, frontal headaches, general frustration or tightness, nervous conditions, mental pressures, constipation, and sexual inhibitions.

Constipation

Constipation is the condition where fecal matter is retained in the large intestine or rectum and not properly excreted. Hard or infrequent bowel movements, gas, abdominal pain, bloating, and headaches can result.

Major Causes

Constipation can be caused by (1) eating devitalized, starchy foods, especially those made with white flour, which do not supply us with enough roughage, (2) eating rich or heavy foods, (3) eating too many kinds of foods at once*, (4) abdominal tension, or (5) lack of exercise. Any one of these conditions can result in waste matter being blocked in the colon.

Health authorities agree that constipation can be prevented by eating properly and getting enough exercise. We are created to have an easy and regular elimination of waste, not to become clogged up.

Live foods such as sprouts, fresh fruits and vegetables, and whole grains all contain healthy roughage which encourages proper elimination. A salad made from fresh spinach, parsley, lettuce, cucumbers, sprouts, bell pepper, and green beans is high in fiber and the Vitamins A, B, C, E, G, and K which help to relieve constipation.[27] Oily seeds, such as flax seeds, and bran are also helpful.

Exercise such as brisk walking (swinging your hands freely by your sides), jogging, swimming, and Acu-Yoga all tone and massage the muscles of the intestinal tract. Daily exercise promotes regularity of the bowels as well as keeping your whole body energized and in good tone.

> *"With regard to our physical health, movement is the principle thing, regulation of movement of its rhythm in pulsation and the circulation of the blood. The whole cause of death and decay is to be traced to the lack of movement; all different aspects of diseases are to be traced to congestion. Every decay is caused by congestion, and congestion is caused by lack of movement."*[28]

Types of Constipation

According to the Chinese, there are four types of constipation: hot, cold, gassy, and bloody.[29]

Hot constipation, a yang condition, can be caused by too much salt or meat, or by a heavily stressful life style. Eating prunes or sour apples and physical exercise may benefit this condition.

---

* Please see section on "Indigestion" for a discussion of food combining.
[27] Mildred Jackson, *The Handbook of Alternatives to Chemical Medicine*, page 52.
[28] Sufi Inayat Khan, *The Book of Health*, page 9.
[29] *A Barefoot Doctor's Manual*, pages 87–88.

Cold constipation, a yin condition, can result from eating an excess of sugar, honey, fruit, juice, or other fluids. The intestinal walls may become weak or bloated, and lose the muscle tone needed for proper peristaltic contraction. The colon needs to be warmed or tonified through abdominal exercise, and through eating more yang foods and fiber foods, such as whole grains.

Gassy constipation, is due to the putrefication of incompletely digested food caught in the large intestine. Traditionally, the Chinese recommend eating less and exercising more for this type of constipation. Raw vegetable salads and sprouted grains also are beneficial.

Bloody constipation, is an extreme condition that requires a doctor's attention. The blood must be nourished and the intestines lubricated. Traditionally, sesame seeds, peach kernels, and herbal teas were given for this type of constipation.

Indicator	Hot	Cold	Gassy	Bloody
Abdomen	Distended, painful	Intermittent pain	Gassy	Distended
Bowels	Hard	No movement	No movement	Stools tarry
Lips	Black	Pale		
Mouth	Dry	Not dry	Belching	Dry
Tongue	Yellow	White	White	Purplish red
Body	Feels hot	Cold hands and feet	Distended	Restless
Urine	Brown	Clear		

Practice the "Knee Squeeze" listed under "Indigestion" on page 188 and this next Acu-Yoga exercise, "Squat Pose," to improve elimination. Squat Pose strongly opens the descending flows. Therefore it is not to be done by pregnant women, who should use diet, exercise, and massage to prevent constipation.

Squat Pose

1. Stand with your feet comfortably apart and lean forward. Grasp the backs of your knees with your hands so that your thumbs are on the outside and fingers on the inside. Your palms will be against the back of your legs with the webbing between the thumb and index finger at the back of the knee.

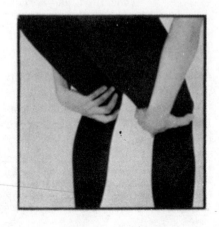

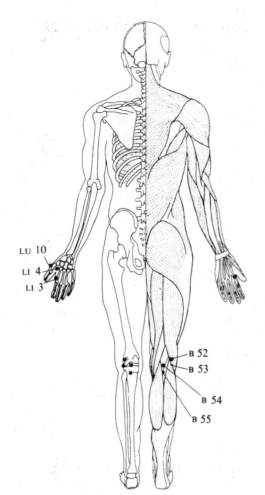

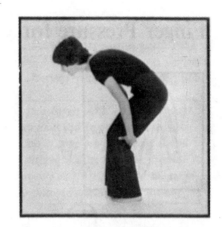

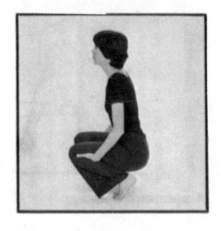

2. Keeping your hands in this position, squat down so that pressure is created on Large Intestine 4, "Hoku," and the rectum has a sensation of openness.

3. Breathe into your belly in this position for one minute.

4. Return to standing and relax.

Acu Points	Traditional Associations
Large Intestine 3, 4	Brings up much mucus, frontal headache, migraine.
Lung 10	Upset stomach, headache, vertigo, insomnia.
Bladder 52, 53	Constipation, lower abdomen hot and hard, abdominal distension, cystitis, muscular spasms in general.
Bladder 54, 55	Lumbago with stiff neck, arthritis of the knee, body feels heavy, bleeding, hemorrhoids, abdominal pain, vaginal spasm.

Benefits: elimination, frontal headaches, muscular spasms in general, hemorrhoids, constipation, abdominal pain.

Finger Pressure for Constipation

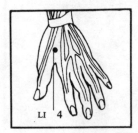

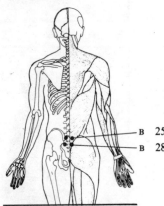

Acupressure Points

The following points have been traditionally used for constipation. Hold each point for several minutes with firm, deep pressure.

● **Large Intestine 4** (Hoku), "The Great Eliminator." Located in the webbing between the thumb and index finger, it is the most famous and widely used point for constipation.

● **Bladder 25** is the Associated Point for the Large Intestine. Located on the lower back on the most prominent knobs of the hip bones beside the fifth, or lowest lumbar vertebra.

● **Bladder 28** is traditionally used for abdominal problems, including constipation. It is located about three fingers width outside the sacroiliac joint on the buttocks.

Acupressure Massage

This routine for constipation can be done either on another person or on oneself. The following are instructions for working on another person; adjustments can be easily made to adapt this to working on yourself.

1. Have the recipient breathe deeply during the entire exercise. Start with the recipient on his or her back, with knees up, feet flat on the floor.

2. Starting at the top of the abdomen, press into the abdominal points located in a circle over the abdomen. Work slowly, moving in a clockwise direction.

3. Knead the entire abdomen with the heel of your hand. Repeat the slow clockwise rotation on the abdominal points, pressing a little more firmly the second and third times around.

4. Have the person turn over and lie on her or his stomach.

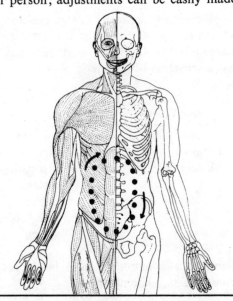

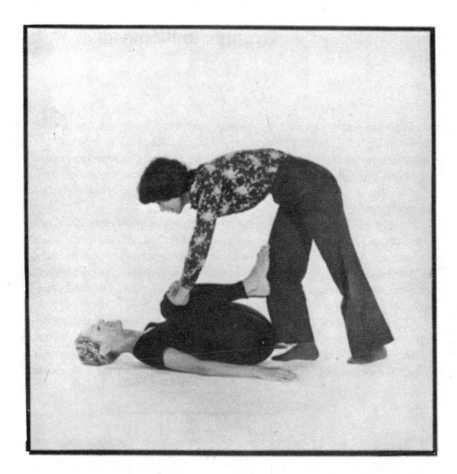

5. Press the points on either side of the spine in the lower back area. Massage the entire buttocks and lower back areas.

6. Have the person turn over and lie on their back again. Bend their legs, pressing the knees together and toward the chest. Keep firm pressure with the heels of your hands on the point just below the knee on the outside of the leg (Stomach 36). Have the recipient breathe long and deep for several minutes.

7. Extend the recipient's legs straight out in front of them. Allow the person to lie on their back and relax for a few minutes.

8. In order to prevent future constipation, encourage the person to exercise daily and eat plenty of fresh vegetables and whole grains.

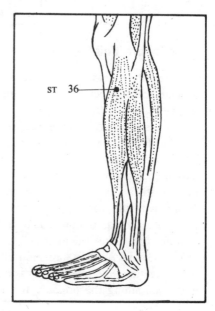

ST 36

Cramps and Spasms

Cramps are usually caused by muscular tension. Tense muscles already in a contracted state inhibit circulation so that lactic acid and other toxins accumulate. This further imbalances the area, causing a stagnation of energy and reinforcing tension. During a cramp the nerves of the affected muscle are hyperactive, causing an extreme and sudden contraction of the muscle, the cramp or spasm. Cramps are an example of an excessively yang (contracted) condition.

Cramps can develop in any muscle in the body, but they usually occur in muscles which have been excessively used, or over trained. Athletes, therefore, tend to develop cramps in the muscles used most, so that pitchers may experience arm or shoulder cramps, and runners may get cramps in their feet or legs. It also happens that muscles used a great deal at one time may develop cramps years later, if muscle tone is not maintained by activity and exercise.

The location of a cramp also relates to the meridian that travels through the affected area. Cramps in the back, and along the backs of the legs are thus associated with the Bladder and Kidney Meridians, and indicate imbalance and excessive tension. Cramps along the sides of the body would similarly be related to the Gall Bladder Meridian.

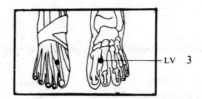

LV 3

Acupressure Points

Acupressure points are keys for releasing muscular cramps in two ways: (1) by using a specific point associated with cramps, and (2) by pressing points directly on the cramped muscle.

The first method uses the Acupressure point Liver 3 for preventing cramps and spasms. It is located on the top of the foot in the valley between the large and second toes (see diagram above). This is the balancing point of the Liver Meridian, and is traditionally associated with cramps and spasms. If you get a cramp, immediately press this point strongly along with a local point in the area of the cramp as instructed in the second method. Prolonged firm pressure on these two points releases the cramp surprisingly quickly. After the cramp has eased, continue to hold Liver 3 and the local point gently for a few more minutes to balance the area.

The second Acupressure method uses a local point for releasing a cramped muscle. This direct method involves pressing very gradually into the heart of the cramped muscle, and maintaining the pressure for about two or three minutes. This prolonged pressure counters the force of the cramp. This illustrates an important principle of yin and yang: when two yang forces oppose one another, one eventually yields to the other. As long as you hold the point with steady, firm pressure, you can "outlast" the force of the cramp, and it will yield to your pressure.

Dietary Considerations

There are also dietary considerations associated with cramps. Foods which tend to constrict and tighten the muscles lay a foundation for potential cramping problems. Meat and salt are the main examples of foods which have a binding and contracting effect on the muscles. When eaten in excess, meat or salt contribute to tension. An excess amount of salt will stiffen the muscles and have an overall rigidifying effect.

Cramps can also be caused by a need for calcium in the muscles. Since Vitamins D and E assist in the assimilation of calcium, it's important to get enough of them. Fresh lemon juice in a glass of warm water, for example, provides the body with these vitamins.[30]

Traditionally, muscle cramps are related to the Liver. Thus Liver 3, discussed above, is an obvious point to use for cramps. According to the classics, the flavor associated with the Liver is sourness. A moderate amount of sour flavored foods in one's diet can improve muscle tone and aid in preventing cramps. Conversely, an excess amount of sour or salty foods can toughen the flesh.[31]

Preventing Cramps

Prevention is the best approach for cramps. Both Acu-Yoga and massage can contribute to keeping the muscles stretched out and flexible, which is the surest way to prevent cramping.

Acu-Yoga helps in two ways. Firstly, it increases your awareness of your muscle tension, so that you know which areas need the most attention. Secondly, practicing the postures stretches, loosens, and relaxes the muscles, thus eroding the tension which is the prerequisite for cramping and spasms. For example, the Bladder Meridian Stretch works on the backs of the calves and thighs.

Massaging tense muscles that tend to cramp up is also helpful. If you have a problem with cramps in a particular area, massage it daily along with the occasional use of hot compresses, which also help relax muscular tension. For example, if your calf muscles tend cramp, knead the entire length of the muscle. Be sure to work on it all the way from the Achilles tendon, above the heel, to the back of the knee. Whenever a muscle feels particularly tense, take 15–20 minutes for massage, stretching, and heat to loosen it up *before* it gets to the point where it will cramp up.

The following exercise, "Yoga Mudra," is often called "baby pose," because infants commonly relax in this position. Yoga Mudra compresses the thorax and abdomen to expel stagnant air out of the lungs. It helps eliminate gas and improve digestion. The associated Acupressure points for this posture have been traditionally used for relieving and preventing cramps, including stomach and menstrual cramps.

---

[30] Mildred Jackson, *The Handbook of Alternatives to Chemical Medicine*, page 68.
[31] Ilza Veith, *The Yellow Emperor's Classic of Internal Medicine*, pages. 21–23.

Yoga Mudra

1. Sit on your heels with your feet spread about two feet apart, and your arms hanging loosely at your sides.

2. Inhale deeply, then exhale and slowly bend forward towards the floor, until your forehead rests on the ground. Your arms are now on the floor by the sides of your body.

3. Now place your hands under your feet so that your index finger is on Liver 3 (in the valley between the big toe and the second toe, about an inch up onto the top of the foot).

4. Breathe deeply in this position. Concentrate on breathing fresh life energy into your muscles, and exhaling toxins and tensions away. Let each breath be slow and complete.

5. Continue for one minute. Gradually work up to two minutes in the pose.

6. Relax on your back for a few minutes, allowing all of the major muscular areas of your body to completely relax.

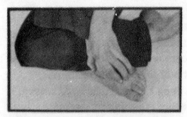

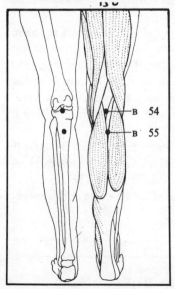

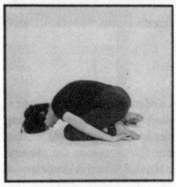

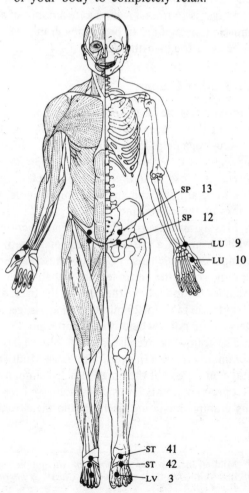

Acu Point	Traditional Associations
Liver 3	Muscular cramps and spasms, liver problems, eyes burning or unclear vision, toes cramping or feet weak, face and eyes pale.
Lung 9, 10	Lung balancing.
Stomach 41	Muscles numb, rheumatism, fear or agitation.
Stomach 42	Walking around aimlessly, seeking warmth.
Spleen 12, 13	Gastric or intestinal spasms, abdominal pain or indigestion.
Bladder 54, 55	Numbness or coldness of lower extremities, spasms, rheumatism, vaginal cramps.

Benefits: indigestion, constipation, gas, rheumatism, angry temper, aggression, hay fever and allergies.

Depression

Depression is an expression that something in our life is lacking or imbalanced. For example, often we get depressed when we lack purpose in our lives. Various neurotic habits are associated with depression. Self-destructive impulses such as smoking, drinking, or overeating, weaken and further imbalance our physical and emotional state. Consequently our morale is lowered and our system partially shuts down. The result is depression.

The darkness of a depression can, however, lead us to the other end of the spectrum, to self-awareness. The key is to be mindful, to be open to a new sense of awareness as a guiding light for changing our lives.

Depression is simply something to work with for discovering more about ourselves. We get off the track when we judge these feelings. Our emotions are simply there for us to learn from as an expression of the moment.

The practice of Acu-Yoga, like most disciplines, can quickly bring us to our inner barriers: "*I can't.*" "*It's too hard.*" "*I don't want to do it anymore.*" "*I don't like this anyway.*" "*This is stupid.*" "*My foot (back, neck, head, stomach, finger, etc.) hurts.*" "*I'm not good enough.*" These are some examples of inner blocks and resistances that we all have.

In addition to these psychological blocks, there are also dietary and physiological causes of depression. The important thing is that we can *choose* to look at all of them. Self-awareness plays a key role in guiding us through the barriers that limit our exploration and growth.

Working with Depression

The points and postures of Acu-Yoga automatically release energies inside us that have been blocked. As the energy flows through the meridians, it opens up blocked parts of the body, and the feelings associated with that blockage rise to the surface. A new awareness of these feelings can then be experienced.

It is up to us. We can choose to observe, accept, and deal with whatever feelings surface. We have the opportunity to play therapist, to step aside a little and look at what's happening. This isn't easy; it is hard work to really look at oneself. We're very used to *not* looking, to blaming someone else when we're upset. It can also be frightening to let go of the defenses that have been "protecting" us from our feelings all these years. Fears, self-doubts, angers that we never knew were inside can surface. If, however, we persist in looking, we can gain an experience of and insight to these feelings and loosen their hold on us. The more it is done, the easier it becomes, and the better we feel deep down inside. If we can listen to whatever comes to the surface from deep inside, we can learn a staggering amount. Our daily thoughts can be an expression of the teacher within.

Psychological Considerations

Depression can result from repressed emotions. Most of us learn from an early age that society requires us to act acceptably by pushing our feelings aside. Because a young child's survival depends upon being accepted, we often repress our feelings and literally *act* in ways that will please others. Unfortunately, we carry these emotional habits with us even after they no longer apply.

There are three main stages for obtaining self-awareness: observation, acceptance, and responsibility. Each level is important for psychological growth.

Observation: The first step of the growth process is simply to observe without judgment. Notice that judgments come up, and observe them also. In Yoga this is traditionally called "witnessing." In the process of observing ourselves when we're upset, we automatically separate ourselves from being the upset. From this more detached vantage point we are better able to examine what's really causing the depression.

Acceptance: The second step is acceptance. After observing, we are free to accept whatever's there without judgments of right/wrong, good/bad, smart/stupid, success/failure, attractive/ugly, superior/inferior, and so on. Often depression stems from judging ourselves to be "bad," and, of course, we are our own harshest critic. This depression can then lead to regret, self-pity, or doubt. If, however, we can get beyond all this by first *observing* and then accepting, depression will fade away because it is no longer fed with the negative emotional energy it needs to survive.

The goal is to accept ourselves exactly as we are: all the things that have happened to us, the ways we have handled our lives, our feelings of how we have been treated, our expectations, hopes, fears, angers, loves, joys, and highest dreams. These are all a part of us. This is simply what is. We can step aside and look at this truth, and simply accept it for what it is.

Responsibility: Ultimately, you are responsible for the experience of your own life, for what in fact you do to yourself. We are the only ones who can choose and control how we treat ourselves. We have the ability to accept and love ourselves just as we are, to take care of and nurture ourselves, and to respond to the inner voices and emotional expressions that constantly come up. It is up to us to take responsibility for how we experience life. And with responsibility comes a freedom and satisfaction in life that seems amazing. This process of unfolding through observation and acceptance to responsibility seems miraculous, but anyone can do it.

The following four aspects are important elements for developing personal fulfillment and for preventing depression.

- *Self-Love*: Choosing to create or cultivate positive situations that fulfill personal needs and promote growth.
- *Mutual Relationships*: Becoming involved with people who are willing to be positive, who share in giving and receiving, and who love.
- *Meaningful Work*: Finding a form of service that contributes to one's purpose and identity.
- *Future Visions*: Visualizing desirable changes in our lives. Making goals and working towards them.

Dietary Considerations

Depression can also be the result of hypoglycemia (low blood sugar), a yin condition where one's feelings tend to fluctuate from extreme highs to extreme lows. Hypoglycemia can be caused by too much sugar in the diet. For a short while the consumption of sugar raises the blood sugar level producing a sort of high. To balance this sharp rise, however, the pancreas produces too much insulin which lowers the blood sugar level too drastically and causes fatigue, depression, or nervousness.

People with hypoglycemia should avoid sugar and other yin substances such as alcohol, coffee, and fruits with a high sugar content. Fresh vegetables, well-chewed whole grains, miso soup, sprouts, and sea vegetables are excellent foods that balance yin conditions.

Depression can also be caused by deficiencies of Vitamin C and E. Parsley-cucumber salads made with fresh lemon juice are a rich source of these vitamins.

Physiological Considerations

Depression can also be the result of an inadequate supply of oxygen in the blood. This can be improved in two ways: first, by strengthening the Spleen Meridian, which is associated with the blood, and second, by deep breathing, which increases the oxygen supply. The spleen is also associated with the pancreas, which, as mentioned previously, is involved in low-blood sugar conditions.

The spleen produces and stores the blood which carries oxygen to the cells of the entire body. When the body needs a greater blood supply, it calls on the spleen.

> *"If the muscles of the spleen contract, as they do in circumstances which evoke action of the sympathico-adrenal system, e.g., whenever there is oxygen-want, they squeeze out the contents. These corpuscles (red blood cells), of course, at once become carriers of oxygen and carbon dioxide, at a time when their services are in demand."*[32]

Spleen 10, an Acupressure point, located about four fingers width above the kneecap on the inner part of the thigh, may be helpful in dealing with depression related to anemic conditions where there is inadequate oxygenation reaching the body's cells. Its traditional name, in fact, is "sea of blood." Spleen 3 and 4, along the inside arch of the foot, are also beneficial for activating the Spleen Meridian.

The breath is the second consideration. When depressed, watch your breath: it will most likely be shallow and constricted. Therefore, a practical, simple, and effective Yogic technique for depression is to increase the depth of the breath. Anybody can come out of a depression (if they really want to, that is) in five minutes by making each breath as long and deep as possible. This sounds simple, but it takes deep concentration. If one increases the depth of one's breath so that four breaths a minute are taken, within five minutes it will *completely* change how one feels about oneself. Try it. The Acu-Yoga exercise described below, "Bringing In and Letting Go," is a breathing exercise that can accomplish this transition.

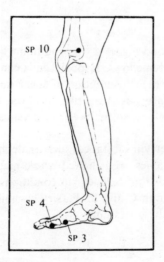

---

[32] Walter Cannon, M. D., *The Wisdom of the Body*, page 166.

Using Acu-Yoga for Depression

Acu-Yoga is a powerful way to develop self-awareness. It enables us to gain a new sense of our bodies and reestablish a connection with the life forces of nature. The postures, points, and breathing open us to that infinite source of energy. As this life force circulates through our meridians, it releases a flow of aliveness, creativity, and awareness. Acu-Yoga's deep breathing exercises can free us from a depression by helping us become more aware of the blocks and energy within. They can also prevent depressions from occurring in the first place.

Life constantly tests us with obstacles and barriers. If we work to build strength, flexibility, balance, and perseverance through a discipline such as Acu-Yoga, we have a foundation against life hitting us with a tough one. By using what we have built, we can turn the "problems" of life into exciting challenges and opportunities for growth.

Bringing In and Letting Go

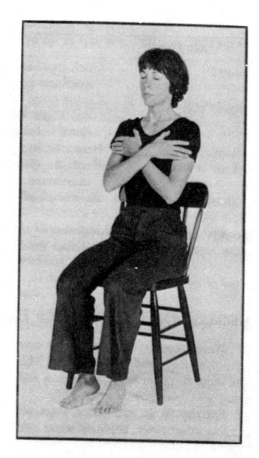

1. Sit comfortably with your spine straight.
2. Cross your arms in front of your chest. Let your fingers contact the upper outside area of the chest, which will probably be tight (Lung 1). Your wrists cross at your "Heart Center."
3. Let your head rest forward (chin towards the hollow at the base of the throat).
4. Inhale four short breaths in a row through your nose, filling your lungs completely on the fourth breath. Hold the breath for a few seconds with the chest full and expanded.
5. Exhale slowly through your mouth.
6. Continue for three minutes, concentrating on the depth and rhythm of the breath.

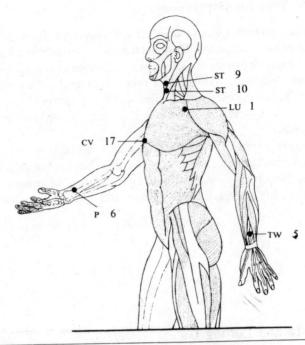

Acu Points	Traditional Associations
Lung 1	Grief, emotional holding, depression, fullness and heaviness in chest, difficult breathing.
Conception Vessel 17	Central point where the Heart, Lung, Spleen, Liver, Kidney, and Triple Warmer Meridians meet; anxiety and emotional imbalances.
Triple Warmer 5	Headache, hypertension, chest pain, depression.
Pericardium 6	Headache, dizziness, madness, insanity, and emotional imbalances.
Stomach 9, 10	Thyroid gland, self-expression.

Benefits: the heart, chest congestion or tightness, instability, worry, self-doubt, excessive anger, lack of courage, emotional imbalance.

Additional Quick Techniques for Depression

1. **Water Therapy:** Run cold water over the ankles, feet, hands, face, and ears. This will stimulate all the meridians to flow and boost your energy.
2. **Exercise:** Walk, run, dance, swim, lift weights, roller skate, anything where you work up a sweat and release some tension.
3. **Self-Expression:** Use a creative outlet to express your feelings. "Sing the Blues," draw, color, paint, or dance your feelings and stumbling blocks. Or write about it —whatever you feel like.

Eye Problems

Eyestrain is mainly caused by (1) cultural, environmental, or occupational conditions which demand overuse of the eyes, or (2) emotional or physical stress. Although eye problems can also be the result of an accident or genetic influence, this section will focus on the cultural, physical, and emotional causes, including practical methods and insights for eye improvement.

Cultural Influences

Many conditions of modern life make us especially susceptible to eyestrain. Firstly, with lighting available at any time of the day or night, we are more likely to spend many more hours using our eyes than we otherwise possibly could. Secondly, the sedentary practice of watching TV and movies for long periods of time can strain the eyes. We sit for hours, with mainly our eyes working and becoming fatigued. Our culture has grown so that we use our eyes much, much more than our other senses. People depend mostly on their vision for work, play, and survival, resulting in overwork for the eyes. Eye problems can result from this dependency.

Even simply the use of electrical lighting itself can strain the eyes, since it is artificial and does not include all the wave-lengths available in sunlight, the type of light our eyes evolved to see by. Additionally, we use our eyes a lot for close work, and spend more and more time indoors, where the range of our vision is limited. The eyes have to work to focus on objects close to us, whereas they relax when looking at things at a distance. Be sure to rest your eyes when reading, watching TV, etc., by frequently looking up for a moment at something in the distance. You can immediately feel your eyes relax.

Emotional Influences

Many types of emotional stress get stored in the eyes. Many people have been taught not to cry, so that their eye muscles are chronically tense, holding back the feelings that have been pushed down inside. Deep internalized stress can actually affect our vision through the state of the nervous system. Our emotions greatly influence the condition of the nerves. If our emotions are imbalanced, stagnant patterns can develop which restrict our visual capabilities, so that we don't see as well as we should.

Another emotional association with the eyes is those experiences that we don't want to see, that we have been taught not to see, or acknowledge. As a child, what images were denied or repressed? Did you emotionally shield your eyes to hide, withdraw, or to protect yourself? Getting in touch with and expressing these buried feelings—repressed fear, anger, sadness—can help reopen our vision. The emotion of anger is especially associated with eye problems or weakness. Also, notice whether you actually look directly at people or not, especially when you're talking to them. Avoiding eye contact can be a way of avoiding your feelings.

The Art of Seeing

Traditionally, the condition of the eyes is associated with the Liver Meridian*. Therefore, by working on this meridian, the eyes can be strengthened and vision improved. The Liver Meridian is related to spring and new green growth. Therefore, fresh green vegetables are good foods for rebalancing this meridian. Avoid eating fatty foods such as meat and dairy products which congest the Liver and have an overall toxic effect on the body.

The eyes are called the "windows of the soul," since they express our inner being, which we can never really hide. The clearer a person is physically, emotionally, and spiritually, the clearer their eyes and their vision of the world.

The way of seeing is an art in itself. The East Indian culture has over 300 words for eye expression. Allow whatever images are there to come, instead of trying to see what you want to see. This is the difference between *looking* and *seeing*.

If a person is looking for something, there is strain and effort. If, on the other hand, one is open to life, trusts the images of the world to enter, and truly accepts what is there, the eyes will be relaxed and the vision clear. Sight can be improved by cultivating this accepting state of mind.

Following are three Acu-Yoga exercises for eye problems: "Eye Circles," "Palming," and "Yoga Mudra."

Eye Circles

1. Sit comfortably with your eyes open.
2. Keeping your eyes open and your head still, look up as far as you can, and then slowly move them in a large circle around the periphery of your vision. Let the movements be slow, smooth, and graceful. Notice any jerkiness, which is a result of tension in the eye muscles.
3. *Slowly* rotate the eyes in this manner for three full circles. Look forward, close your eyes, and relax them.
4. Open your eyes and rotate them in a complete circle three times in the other direction. Then look forward, close your eyes, and relax them.
5. Repeat the entire exercise, three circles in each direction.
6. Close your eyes and relax them for a few minutes, breathing long and deep. The next exercise, "palming," is especially beneficial to practice next.

Palming

1. Sit comfortably and close your eyes. For this exercise you may either wish to sit at a table, resting your elbows on the table, or kneel, resting your elbows on the ground.
2. Fit the heels of your hands over your

---

* This is why anger, which is the emotion related to the Liver Meridian, is especially connected to eye weakness.

eyes. The palms should contact the entire ridge around the eyes. This presses several Acupressure points that directly benefit the eyes.

3. Breathe long and deep. Let your neck, face, and eyes relax fully for a couple of minutes.

4. Remove your palms and slowly open your eyes, maintaining the relaxation. Feel your eyes open, clear and relaxed.

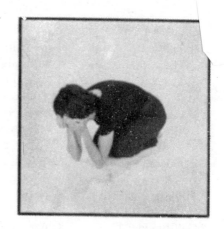

Yoga Mudra

1. Kneel with your large toes touching each other, heels apart, and your arms hanging loosely at your sides.

2. Inhale deeply, then exhale and slowly bend forward, bringing your elbows to your thighs, a few inches above your knees.

3. Make your hands into fists and raise your head slightly, placing your fists on the floor—so that your head will rest on them. The knuckles of the index and middle fingers are placed so that the ridge of the eye (Bladder 1 and 2) rests between them.

4. Breathe deeply in this position. Consciously relax your eyes, and visualize a black velvet screen. Allow yourself to see whatever images come up for you.

5. Continue for one or two minutes.

6. Sit comfortably or lie down and rest for a few minutes.

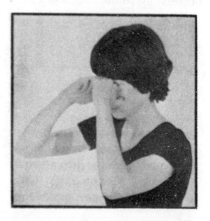

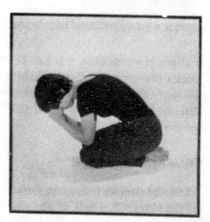

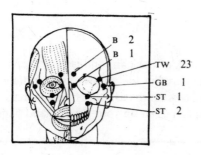

Acu Point	Traditional Associations
Stomach 1 "Receive Tears"	Poor vision, eyes twitch and water, dislike of strong light, poor night vision.
Stomach 2 "Four Whites"	Eyes feel dizzy, blink, water easily, feel as if they have smoke in them. Facial tension.
Bladder 1 "Eyes Bright"	Master point for the eyes. Eyes dizzy, white membrane over eyes, tears flow in wind, dim vision, poor night vision, conjunctivitis.
Bladder 2 "Drilling Bamboo"	Eyes red, painful, lazy, wandering, watering. Excessive blinking, vision foggy, headache, hallucinations.
Triple Warmer 23 "Bamboo Hollow"	Eyes red, swollen, painful, twitch, blink excessively, tearing and inflammation in bright light, vision blurred.
Gall Bladder 1 "Eye Born"	Outer corners of eyes red and painful. Weak eyesight, color blindness.

Benefits: eyestrain, liver and gall bladder imbalances, neck tension, nervous disorders.

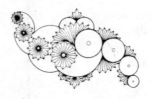

Fatigue

Fatigue is a condition that can be caused by various imblances, including physical deficiencies and excesses, dietary habits, emotional problems, and stagnant mental outlooks. By working on yourself on different levels you can begin to reverse the processes that cause fatigue. You can free yourself to experience both short and long-range improvements in your vitality.

Physical Deficiencies

Three deficiencies that cause fatigue are (1) a lack of fresh air, and lack of deep ventilation of the lungs; (2) a lack of the vital Ki energy through the points and meridians; and (3) inadequate circulation of the blood. Muscular tension in various degrees increase all these problems. By *releasing* tension, however, you can open up your system, and begin to free yourself from fatigue.

The Breath

Many people spend a lot of their time indoors, both at work and at home, and therefore get very little fresh air. Even if you live in an area that suffers from air pollution, it is better to get outside at least some time during the day to get away from the stagnant, and often dried-out indoor air.

How you breathe is important, as well as *what* you breathe. Tight chest muscles constrict the ribs so that they cannot work properly; many people breathe only shallowly. When this tension begins to be released, however, the chest can open the lungs more completely, resulting in deep, full breathing, and a greater oxygenation of the blood.

Many people only take deep breaths when they yawn, by which time they're *already* fatigued! Yawning is a reflex action whereby the body *forces* a deep breath to exhale stale air and get more oxygen to the blood. If you're not sure how deep or shallow your breathing is, take a yawn and feel how long and deep a breath it makes. Is yawning the only way *you* usually breathe deeply?

If so, deeper breathing alone can greatly increase your energy level, and can also help you relax. Many people are on a seesaw between pushing themselves and collapsing with fatigue. It's wonderful to begin the process of replacing these negative extremes with a harmonious balance of activity and relaxation. You may wish to refer to the section on "Deep Breathing" for a more complete discussion.

Ki Energy*

The Chinese traditionally believe that we are born with a certain amount of Ki energy, the amount depending generally on the state of health of our parents, and even of our ancestors. Further, we can either retain that inherited energy, deplete it, or increase it through the way we live. Factors that affect the level of our Ki energy are eating, exercise, and breathing habits; mental and emotional conditions; deleterious habits, such as smoking, drinking, and taking drugs; and environmental conditions, such as air quality and noise pollution.

When this energy is depleted by unhealthy living habits, there is less vital energy flowing through the Acupressure points and meridians. This in turn has a negative effect on the internal organs, and lowers our resistance to disease in general.

But when we work to build up a strong Ki energy reserve, we can strengthen and revitalize our organs, as well as our overall resistance. We can accomplish this through good diet, exercise, deep breathing, Acupressure and Acu-Yoga. Other methods, such as the Oriental art of Tai Chi Chuan, also build Ki energy reserves.

Circulation

Poor circulation can result in undernourishment of the cells and tissues, since the nutrients in the blood cannot reach the cells as fully as possible and the toxic by-products of cell metabolism cannot be completely carried away and excreted. Stagnation and tension in the area are the result.

Muscular tension decreases circulation of both the blood and the Ki energy, and blocks deep breathing. It's wonderful to experience the process of unblocking muscular armor, and the expansion of health and vitality that results from this process.

---

* Ki is the life energy that circulates throughout the human body.

Conditions of Excess

Excesses, as well as deficiencies, can cause a lack of energy. Many people tend to push themselves too hard, to end up "running on nervous energy." But you can only push yourself so far before you snap. We aren't built to withstand more than a certain amount of stress. We each have to determine for ourselves how much is too much. Everybody has different stress limitations and overload levels. When you tune in to yourself and cultivate your inner awareness, you can discover what is your optimum balance of activity and rest.

Traditionally, the Chinese discovered that excesses of particular activities weaken particular Acupressure meridians:

- Excess standing damages the Kidney Meridian
- Excess sitting damages the Spleen Meridian
- Excess lying down damages the Lung Meridian
- Excess looking damages the Heart Meridian
- Excess physical exertion damages the Liver Meridian

You might want to work on points, for example on the Kidney Meridian, if you have to stand up a lot. Many occupations demand that people do an excessive amount of standing, sitting, or using the eyes. It's important to counteract these stresses in order to prevent fatigue.

Techniques for Relieving Fatigue

Foot Massage

Foot massage is an excellent way of overcoming fatigue and restoring vitality. Take off your shoes and socks. Firmly massage the ankles and the arches of both feet. Next massage the soles of the feet and the toes. Half of the organ meridians run through the feet, especially through the toes.

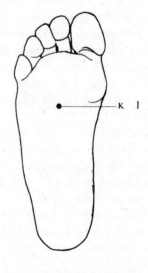

When you massage your feet be sure to work on Kidney 1, the first point on the Kidney Meridian, located on the sole at the bottom of the ball of the foot (see diagram). This point, called "Bubbling Spring," is an Acupressure first-aid revival point. It's a source of energy for the entire body, and provides a quick way to pick yourself up from a state of fatigue.

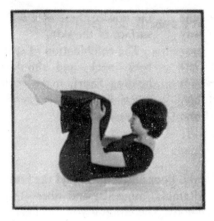
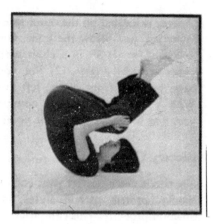

Spinal Rocking

Rocking on your spine is another easy technique for relieving fatigue, and one that works on different aspects of the body. First, of course, it provides a good massage for the spine, the back muscles, and all the Acupressure points that run alongside the spine. All the nerves stemming out of the spine are related to all the organs, as are the Acupressure points on the spinal muscles, so rocking on the spine is actually a whole-body treatment.

Secondly, spinal rocking works on tension in the neck and shoulder area, which can also cause fatigue. By rocking all the way up onto your shoulders and neck you press the muscles and points there, releasing tightness.

Thirdly, during the spinal rocking the hands are placed on a specific Acupressure point, Stomach 36. This point has certain traditional associations: it helps strengthen all the muscles, and is the most widely used point for revitalizing the whole body.

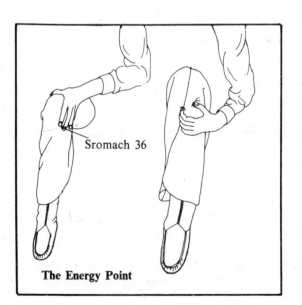

Sromach 36

The Energy Point

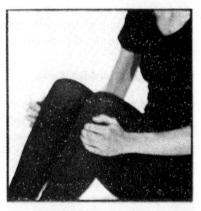

Stomach 36 is called "Sanri," which means "Three More Miles." Its muscle strengthening qualities work for greater endurance. Athletes, hikers, and backpackers can use this strong Acupressure point as a tonic to release physical fatigue.

Sanri is located on the outer side of the lower leg, just below the knee. One way to find it is: (1) Sit in a chair with your knees at right angles. (2) Put your left palm over the front of the left knee. (3) With your fingers spread comfortably, your ring finger will be on the point. Press the muslce there at a 90° angle from the surface of the skin.

The combination of stimulating various back, neck, and shoulder points while holding Sanri, makes spinal rocking an especially effective exercise for physical rejuvenation.

Dietary Considerations

The foods you eat affect your energy level. Poor nutrition starves the body of the building blocks—protein, carbohydrates, fat, vitamins, minerals, and fiber—that it requires to function properly. This can fatigue the body. Therefore, if you *don't* eat nourishing food, and *do* eat items that actively detract from health and well-being, you shouldn't be surprised if you have a problem with lack of energy.

Salt and sugar, for example, are two substances which many people consume excessively. Processed foods usually contain one or the other, if not both. Salt and sugar both can cause fatigue by creating biochemical imbalances. Sugar depletes the body of vitamins, and strains the pancreas, which has a more difficult job of balancing the blood sugar level when sugar is eaten. Salt throws off the body's water balance so that more water is required, but more is also retained in the body. Salt also tends to have a binding or constricting effect on the muscles.

Another dietary problem related to fatigue is overeating, or eating heavy, rich foods. This puts a strain on the digestive system, since it takes extra energy to cope with the overload, thus depleting your available energy. And when your internal organs are tired, so are you.

Fatigue can also be a symptom of overall nutritional deficiencies—of vitamins, minerals, or protein, for example. By eating fresh, unprocessed, and easily digestible foods, however, you can create healthy, well-nourished internal organs. For a more complete discussion of diet, turn to the section on "Indigestion."

Emotional Considerations

A lack of energy can also indicate emotional imblances. If you repress your feelings, you create muscle tention and tightness (in order to literally "hold the lid on"), and you also deaden your experience of your life.

One way you can begin to unblock yourself is through visualization, by opening your mind and imagination. Many people avoid their feelings, thereby deadening themselves, so that their lives are dull and boring.

You can begin to turn boredom around, however, by using your imagination to explore various possible way of being and doing new things. You can open yourself to a new sense of vitality and fulfillment; you can begin to get in touch with deep feelings about what you need and want in life; you can visualize what you want to happen and create a new reality; you *can make* your dreams come true.

This is a part of developing Yogic power through opening the Sixth Chakra, also known as the Third Eye. Visualizations contain an exciting potential for enabling you to expand yourself and your experience of life. The last two exercises in the section on *Chakras* contain visualization techniques that can help you begin to develop this potential.

Mental Considerations

Our minds have tremendous power to influence our lives—more than we are usually led to believe. What we perceive, what we visualize or project to a large extent determines what we get. Our thoughts create our reality by creating *how we perceive* reality.

In this context, it's possible to see how our minds can create fatigue. For example, we may wake up feeling refreshed, but when we look at the clock and see that we got only seven hours of sleep instead of our usual eight we may then feel tired. Fatigue can also be a mental response to do something we don't want to do. The following quite explains other instances of mentally-created fatigue:

> *"Tiredness is geared to three causes: loss of energy, which is the chief reason, and besides this, excess of activity of mind and of body. One generally knows tiredness to be caused by excess of bodily activity, but one is apt to overlook the fact that excess of activity of the mind also causes tiredness.*
>
> *The activities that especially caused tiredness are worry, fear, anxiety, and pain. There is, however, one mental cause that is less obvious, and that is the thought of being tired. Among a hundred cases of tired people you will find 90 cases of this particular kind of tiredness. When a person thinks 'I am tired,' the very thought creates the feeling of tiredness in support of the thought, and the reason brings forward a thousand reasons that seem to have caused the tiredness. There are some who think that the presence of people, or of some people, or the presence of a particular person tires them; some think that their energy, their life, is eaten up by some people; some think that a particular action takes away their energy; some think that strength is taken out of them by their every day duties in life or by the work they happen to do, such as singing, speaking, doing bodily or mental work; and of course, as they think, so they experience."*[33]

The following exercise, "Upholding Heaven with the Two Hands," helps relieve fatigue. It is particularly effective for releasing shoulder tensions. Although it is usually practiced standing up, an advanced version is done on the floor.

---

[33] Sufi Inayat Khan, *The Book of Health*, pages 56–57.

Upholding Heaven with the Two Hands

Standing Position

1. Stand with your feet comfortably apart with your arms at your sides. Your eyes are open during this exercise.
2. Inhale, raising your arms, palms up, out to the sides, all the way up straight above your head.
3. Interlock your fingers with your palms facing down. Rotate your hands so that your palms face the sky. Inhale more and stretch further upwards looking at your hands.
4. Exhale lowering your chin down towards your chest and let your arms float back down to your sides.
5. Repeat five times.

Floor Position (an advanced version)

1. Kneel on the floor. If possible, spread your lower legs apart and sit between them.
2. Supporting yourself with your elbows,

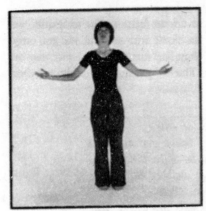

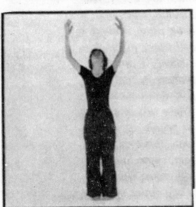

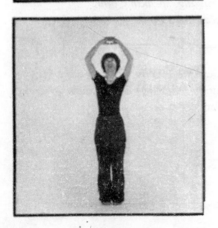

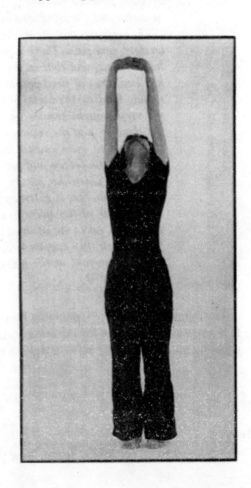

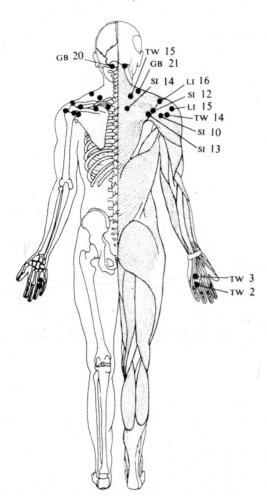

GB 20
TW 15
GB 21
SI 14
LI 16
SI 12
LI 15
TW 14
SI 10
SI 13
TW 3
TW 2

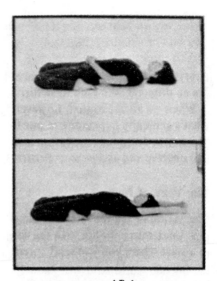

slowly lean back until your upper back and head are on the floor. Your arms are by your sides.

3. Bring your hands to your abdomen and interlace your fingers.

4. Inhale, rotate your hands so that your palms are away from your body, and stretch your arms up and all the way over your head. Stretch your arms fully.

5. Exhale, and slowly let your arms return to the abdomen.

6. Repeat five times. Then come out of the pose and lie flat on your back with your arms at your sides. Relax and feel the energy you've generated.

Acu Points	Traditional Associations
Gall Bladder 20, 21	Arms and shoulder pains, unable to raise hands to the head, rheumatism.
Large Intestine 15, 16	Associated with the shoulder bone and brachial neuralgia.
Triple Warmer 2, 3	Hands or arms red or swollen, fingers cramped, forearm and elbow painful.
Triple Warmer 14, 15	Shoulder and arm painful and cannot move.
Small Intestine 10, 12, 13, 14	Fatigue, stiff neck, muscular pain or weakness in the shoulder and scapula region.

Benefits: fatigue, hypertension, shoulder and neck tensions, rheumatism, arm pain, circulation, emotional or physical cravings, general weakness or a lack of energy.

Frustration

Everything happens at its own pace. Every flower and tree matures at its own rhythm. We are no different. We each have distinctly individual patterns of change and development.

When we are frustrated, however, we are not flowing with our feelings, needs, and with what's generally happening in our lives, but are pushing or resisting something in our life. The key to dropping frustration is to see the truth of these statements, be able to step aside and observe and accept your frustration, and see it as part of a whole.

The Way of Nature

The nature of the universe is change. The next time you feel frustrated or low, remember this. Look into your life with the wisdom that "all things change." When you have evolved to a state where you feel truly interconnected with your environment and the dynamics of the outside world, you will *know* this truth without question. For starters, however, you can simply *pretend* that all things are interconnected and change continuously.

The internal stress behind our frustrations tends to cloud our awareness and faith in the natural dynamics of change. Frustration tends to distort our relative perspective of life. If things have changed to a low or difficult point, they *must* come back up. Life moves in cycles of up and down; it is not stagnant.

Dealing with Obstacles

Many times we perceive situations or aspects of our life as obstacles, and we become frustrated. An obstacle, however, is simply another aspect of life, and is usually our next challenge, the next thing we need to break through to keep expanding and growing. If you become frustrated, step aside from it for a moment and observe what's going on. Is an obstacle involved? Examine it and see what it means to you, how it represents ways you hold yourself back ("*I can't*," "*I don't want to*," "*I'm not good, smart, talented, or rich enough*," "*It's too hard*," etc.).

See that the obstacle is only one aspect of your life, and that there are alternatives and choices surrounding you. You can't see these when you become fixated on or overwhelmed by your obstacle when you just see the problem, and nothing else. Letting go allows other possibilities to come in.

Sometimes you may want to simply accept the obstacle to "put it on hold" for the time being, and other times you may want to work through it. Follow your intuition, and do what feels right to you.

Our limits are continually tested. If you can perceive a frustrating experience as a test, you transform it from an upset to an opportunity and a challenge for growth.

Areas of Muscular Tension

Frustration collects in the body mainly in the shoulders, neck, Solar Plexus, and hips. Through Acu-Yoga, especially the exercises that work on these areas, frustrations can be released. Breathe deeply into your belly, totally putting all of your concentration into the breath. Feel all the motions of your respiratory system: the air in the nostrils, throat, and chest; the belly and chest rising, and the rib cage expanding out to the front, back, and sides. By moving your attention from your emotions to the breath, you can more easily observe and accept things as they are.

The Shoulders can represent uptightness, irritability, fear and resistance to change.

The Solar Plexus is related to the expression of your personal power. Tensions in this area can be a result of the fear of being yourself, a resistance to accepting your power, and being recognized for it. This represents some repression or restriction in your life.

Rigidity in the Neck is associated with anger. Frustrations are a "pain in the neck." Repressed anger creates tension as you jam your feelings down your throat instead of expressing what you want to say.

The Hips also express frustration. People standing with their hands on their hips are often feeling frustrated. They are also instinctually holding Acupressure points related to that frustration. Many important meridians run through the hips, and blockages are common. Starting when children are taught to block out their sexual feelings, to not touch themselves "down there," tension develops in the hips.

The opposite of frustration is well-being, being "in the flow" with things, harmony and aliveness. Frustration is a slow process of death that can be released through movement, which is aliveness. All physical activity can help drain frustrations.

"Movement is life and stillness is death; for in movement there is the significance of life and in stillness we see the sign of death."[34]

The following exercises, "Side Rolls" and "Frustration Release," work especially on the hips to help release tension and frustration.

Side Rolls

1. Lie on your back.
2. Interlace your hands under your neck.
3. Inhale and bend your left leg up.
4. Exhale and roll on your right side, releasing a deep sigh (Ahhhhh).
5. Inhale as you return to lying on your back.
6. Continue for two minutes, alternating sides. Then relax on your back.

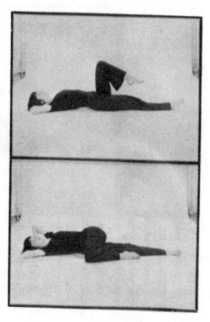

---

[34] Sufi Inayat Khan, *The Book of Health*, page 9.

Acu Points	Traditional Associations
Gall Bladder 30	Frustration, hip problems.
Gall Bladder 20	Frightening, fighting attitude.
Bladder 10	Body relaxant.
Stomach 10	Hypertension.

Benefits: sciatica, headaches, pressure at the base of the skull, low back stiffness.

Frustration Release

1. Lie on your back. Place your hands (or fists) under your buttocks, facing down.
2. Bend your knees and bring your feet comfortably apart.
3. Take a deep breath. On the exhale, move your knees to one side, toward the floor. Your knuckles should be pressing into the central muscles on the buttocks in this position.
4. Inhale as the knees come back to center.
5. Continue for one or two minutes, alternating sides.
6. Relax on your back.

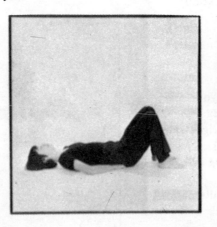
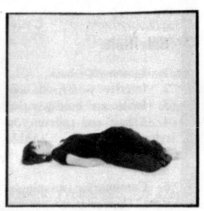

Acu Points	Traditional Associations
Bladder 48	"Womb and Vitals," constipation, heavy feeling pressing downwards.
Bladder 49	Lumbar, sacral pain, urination difficult.
Gall Bladder 30	Buttocks or upper thighs painful, sciatica.

Headaches

Headaches are primarily caused by tension in the muscles of the head, neck, and shoulders. This tension partially constricts the blood vessels that supply the required oxygen to the nerve cells of the brain.

> *"There are important nerve cells in the brain which, if totally deprived of oxygen for more than eight minutes, undergo such profound destructive changes that they do not recover."*[35]

Headaches are an important warning signal of tension and possible oxygen deprivation. They serve as a safety valve to signal our attention to the imbalance in the area before the constriction reaches a critical threshold. Unfortunately, most people choose to repress this signal by taking aspirin, instead of releasing the muslce tension related to the headache. By taking the aspirin they are simply repressing the symptom, instead of dealing with the cause. Once the symptom is repressed, the person is cut off from the body's natural warning mechanisms.

Every symptom we have represents a deeper imbalance in us. Tension headaches derive from the pressures of tight, constricted muscles. Taking a pill to relieve a symptom is a superficial way of dealing with the problem. This example represents the differences between Western and Eastern approaches to health care. Often people tend to avoid many of their body signals (i.e., emotions, minor aches and pains) until they develop into severe conditions that cannot be ignored, and require surgery and other extreme measures. At that point, the disease is dealt with by cutting out the deteriorated organ or part of the body.

The emphasis of traditional Chinese health care is on preventing illness in the first place. The underlying cause of the illnesses that do develop are dealt with in depth, not just by treating superficial symptoms. Symptoms are considered an expression of the condition of the person as a whole. The Eastern ancient doctors went beyond the prevention and treatment of disease to the development of an active, radiant health, for obtaining longevity and enlightenment.

Common Causes of Headaches

- **Emotional Stress:**
  Frustration, anger, worry, fear, and irritability all put a strain on the shoulder, neck, and head muscles, causing pressures and tensions that can lead to headaches.
- **Shoulder and Neck Tension:**
  As mentioned above, pressure in the shoulder and neck muscles directly affects the head area and can partially block the circulation of blood and the flow of vital life energy to the head. This stagnation can result in headaches.
- **Meridian Imbalances:**
  Tension in the head is related to the meridians that flow over it. These include the

---

[35] Walter Cannon, M.D., *The Wisdom of the Body*, page 145.

Gall Bladder (probably the most important, since it zigzags all over the skull), Liver, Triple Warmer, Bladder, and Governing Vessel.

Pressing firmly on the most painful points on the head or face for several minutes can provide effective relief of various headaches. There are also points on the foot (GB 41 and 43, B 62, 64, 67) which help relieve imbalances in these meridians. Gall Bladder 39, located one hand's width above the ankle bone on the outside of the lower leg, is a very strong point for relieving headaches.

● **Cervicial Misalignment:**

If the vertebrae of the neck are out of alignment they throw off the position of the head, creating a strain on neck and head muscles. Discs may be affected so that a neck nerve becomes "pinched," which causes headaches.

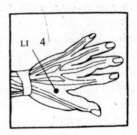

● **Intestinal Congestion:**

Headaches can often be accompanied by constipation.* The point, Large Intestine 4 ("Hoku"), located in the webbing between the thumb and index fingers, helps relieve congestion in both the head and digestive system. Pressing this point alone relieves many headaches temporarily. You then need to look at your diet and see what you can do to unclog your digestive system. Overeating may also cause intestinal congestion. This type of headache usually centers around the forehead or sinus area. Exercising and eating more lightly can help.

Abdominal massage also benefits both constipation and headache. Press points in a circle three inches from the navel (picture a clock, and press one point for each number on the clock). Work in a clockwise direction (facing the abdomen).

● **Dietary Imbalances:**

An excess of salt or sugar—both widely found in modern processed foods—can cause headaches**. They cause gross imbalances in the system when taken in excess. Salt has a contracting effect that accentuates tension. Sugar has a toxic, expanding effect that can cause throbbing in the head. The toxicity of meats can also contribute to cause headaches.

● **Pathological Disease:**

A headache can be a symptom of a more serious condition, such as earache, toothache, rheumatism, or even hemorrhaging or tumors. Again, it acts as a warning signal, and the problem should be brought to a doctor's attention.

---

* See page 143 for the section on "Constipation."
** See page 181 for the section on "Indigestion."

Using Acupressure for Headaches

Shiatsu Techniques

Have the recipient sit comfortably on a stool or use a pillow on the floor.

Stay on the left side of the recipient. Place your right thumb into the medulla oblongata, the hollow in the base of the skull. Support the forehead with your left hand. Rotate the thumb clockwise as you press into the hollow and up underneath the base of the skull. Gradually begin to move the head around. Securely support the head with both hands in this position encouraging the recipient's neck muscles to relax as the head slowly goes around in a wide circular motion.

Next place the back of your fist on the shoulder closely against the neck. Hold the forehead with your other hand, bending the recipient's head back towards the fist. Maintain the position, as illustrated, for approximately 10 seconds. Gradually release the pressure and repeat the move on the other side. This, along with the next technique, is helpful for migraine headaches. Make sure to apply the pressure gradually. It should feel good . . . somewhere between releasing pain and pleasure.

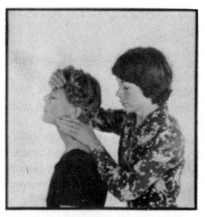

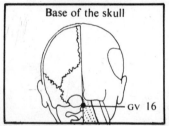

Base of the skull

GV 16

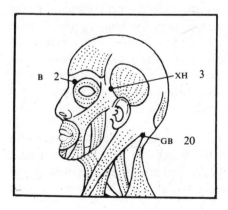

B 2   XH 3

GB 20

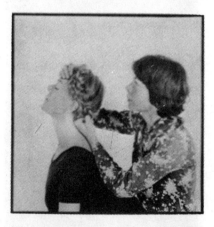

Turn your thumbs up under the occipital bone at the base of the skull. Tilt the recipient's head back a little while you firmly stretch the head straight up, pressing GB 20, underneath the base of the skull. This point is many times the root of headaches. It is sometimes called "the gates of consciousness" for it contributes to regulate the sensorial and neurological activities of the brain.

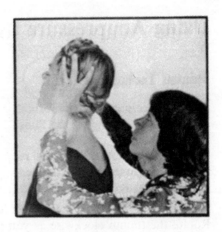

Jin Shin Acupressure

The recipient lies on their back

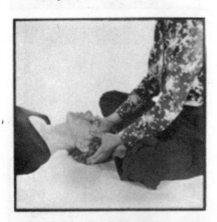

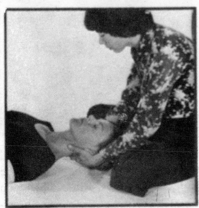

Place your thumbs on the temples (XH 3). Feel for a slight cove where your thumbs seem to fit. Rotate them slowly in a circle. This will gently stretch the skin in this area to relax the auricularis superior muscles. The fingers, instead of the thumbs, can be used to make these circular movements at the temporal region, if you prefer. Afterwards sensitively massage all parts of the ear. This especially benefits the kidneys. There are over a hundred points on the ear which correspond to every part of the body.

Sitting in front of the recipient's head, place both hands underneath the neck. Slowly massage the neck muscles, gently squeezing them by bringing the thumbs and fingers together. Concentrate on squeezing out the greatest tightnesses on the neck. Watch the facial expressions of the recipient as a guide to give you instant feedback.

Then use both of your four fingers to hold the muscles of the back of the neck firmly for a couple of minutes. Release the pressure very slowly. Then scoop the head up in your palms with your fingers curved underneath the base of the skull. Pull the head towards you with the head tilted back, stretching the cervical vertebrae. This will allow the cerebral spinal fluid to circulate into the brain. Release the traction gradually inviting a pulse to come into your finger tips. Hold the base of the skull with your fingers curved until a pulse comes. It should take four minutes at the most. The pulse indicates that energy is circulating through the point (GB 20) into the face and brain.

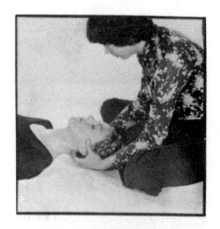

Hold your left hand over the back of the neck with the thumb on the left, fingers on the right for support. Place the four fingers of your right hand over the origins of the eyebrows. There are Acupressure points near the intersection of the eyebrows and the bridge of the nose. These points (B 2) on the ridge of the skull just above the inside of the eye have been traditionally used for minor frontal tension headaches as well as sinus conditions.

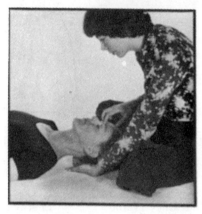

The following two Acu-Yoga exercises, "Looking Under Water" and "Extending the Bridge," help release tensions associated with headaches. Working on specific Acupressure points,* as mentioned in this section, is also beneficial.

Looking Under Water

1. Lie on your stomach with your forehead on the floor. Spread your feet one foot apart.
2. Place your hands behind your head so that you're pressing the points at the base of the skull with your fingers. Your elbows remain resting on the floor.
3. Inhale, raising your head, arms, and feet about three inches off the floor. Press

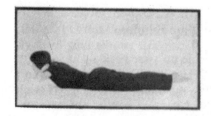

---

* Please refer to "Squat Pose" on page 144.

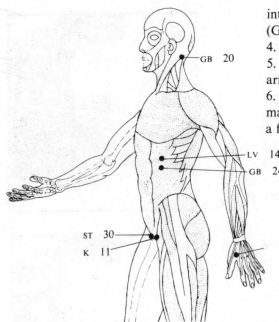

into the base of your skull with your fingers (GB 20).

4. Breathe long and deep for one minute.

5. Relax down, head to one side and arms by your sides.

6. Turn over on your back. Briskly massage "Hoku" (LI 4) and your feet for a further release.

Acu Points	Traditional Associations
Large Intestine 4	Frontal headaches, sinus blockage.
Gall Bladder 20	Migraine headache, eyes hurt, fuzzy thinking.
Gall Bladder 24 and Liver 14	Indigestion, headache.
Kidney 11 and Stomach 30	Energy raises to the top of the body, lower abdomen swollen or painful, cannot stand for long periods of time.

Benefits: abdominal pain, impotency, hernia, penis and scrotum pain, lower backache, headache, bladder weaknesses, urethritis.

In this next exercise, there are two ways to hold the hands. Practice both for the greatest benefit.

Drilling Bamboo

1. Lie on your back.

2. Place your index fingers at the point where the top of the nose meets the inside top of the eye sockets (Bladder 2). The third fingers rest between the brows at the Third Eye, and the thumbs hold the jaw muscles (Stomach 6) or the temples.

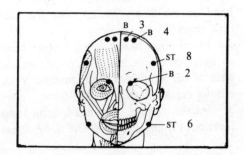

3. Tilt your head all the way back so that your shoulders press up into the base of the skull. Breathe long and deep in this position for about 30 seconds.

4. Then rotate your hands so that your thumbs hold the points the index fingers have been pressing (Bladder 2). Mold your other fingers on the sore points along the hairline. Continue to breathe deeply in this position for about another 30 seconds.

5. Completely relax on your back with your eyes closed.

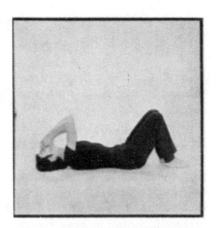

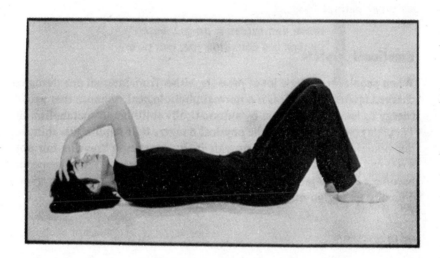

Acu Points	Traditional Associations
Bladder 2	"Drilling Bamboo," brain tired, sinusitis, headache, eyes tired, hay fever.
Bladder 3 and 4	Headache, nose blocked, burning heat in head, eyes tired.
Stomach 6	Facial paralysis, jaw and neck tension, ache.
Stomach 8	"Head Tired," headaches, pain above eyelids.

Benefits: shoulder tension, uptightness, sinus problems, jaw tightness, frontal headaches.

Hypertension

Hypertension, the technical term for high blood pressure, can be caused by dietary imbalances or emotional stress. Various extremes or excesses of these factors can cause or contribute to hypertension.

Regarding dietary factors, there are tension-producing foods and tension-releasing foods. Eating a lot of salt, for example, has been shown to be directly related to high blood pressure. It hardens and constricts the arteries, impeding the blood flow. Thus, the heart must pump harder to circulate the blood through the restricted vessels. Salt tends to stiffen the muscles, creating muscular tensions which also hamper the blood flow. Meat, which contains both salt and animal fats, contributes to hypertension. Since virtually all packaged, canned, processed foods contain salt or white sugar (often both!), they should be avoided. These should be replaced by fresh vegetables and fruits, whole grains, and various other natural foods.

Emotional Aspects

When people are under a lot of pressure, either from internal or external conflicts, they get charged up for action. This is a normal physiological response that provides us with extra energy to handle a situation by automatically shifting our metabolism into a higher gear. These days we aren't facing the physical dangers that require this shift, but unfortunately, our bodies still automatically provide it. By constantly "revving our motors," emotional stress can wear us out. Since a state of high blood pressure is one element in the shift, it can become a chronic problem if we are constantly under a lot of stress, especially if we have difficulty letting go of these pressures.

Hypertension is a symptom, a manifestation of imbalances in the body. Whether dietary or emotional factors predominate, we must look deeply into ourselves and our lives, going beyond symptoms, and looking for causes.* Hypertension can never be completely eliminated until the underlying cause is handled. Holistic health involves looking at ourselves as integrated wholes, and looking beyond symptoms for underlying causes, imbalances and patterns of weakness. In order to achieve radiant health, you must take responsibility to change whatever aspect of your life is causing your imbalances. This can involve changes in your diet, exercise, or work habits. It can mean getting individual help from practitioners of Holistic Health methods. It also requires you to work on yourself, through self-help methods such as meditation and Acu-Yoga. The following story illustrates all of these aspects of hypertension from a holistic perspective.

I used to give Acupressure sessions to a successful and wealthy man who had a bad case of high blood pressure. One time, he relaxed so deeply that he fell asleep for a few minutes so that his session ended a little later than usual. However, he had a doctor's appointment

---

* Please see "Meditation for Exploring the Cause of Disease" on page 44.

soon after that, which he had neglected to tell me about. When he woke he realized he'd be late and started frantically rushing around to get ready.

The Acupressure session had lowered his blood pressure, but I was sure that it had soared back up again from all his rushing around. The next time I spoke with him I was surprised to hear that his doctor said that he had had a normal blood pressure reading for the first time in years.

Blood pressure is one of the few medical tests that I had access to that could measure the benefits of Acupressure. Consequently, I had my client's wife take his blood pressure before and after the Acupressure session so that we could measure the difference. His systolic blood pressure was 162 mm before I worked on him—over 40 mm above normal, which is about 120 mm. After the one-hour session, it had dropped 38 mm to 124 mm.

Even though Acupressure clearly lowered my client's blood pressure, it is only a limited temporary measure unless he looks into what is causing his condition, and begins to deal with that. For example, he had been drinking to "help himself relax." He decided to stop drinking for awhile because he thought he was going to have a heart attack if he didn't, and he was also learning new, constructive ways to relax through Acupressure. His hypertension actually vanished as soon as he stopped drinking.

In the following Acu-Yoga exercise on the next page, "Wing Lifting," points in the shoulders are stretched to release muscle tension and emotional uptightness that contribute to hypertension.

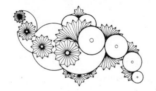

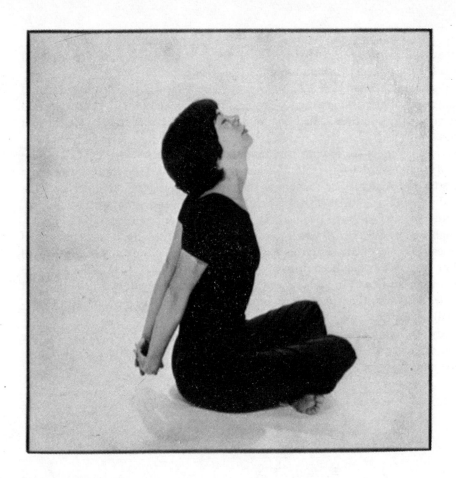

Wing Lifting

1. Sit comfortably and clasp your hands behind your back with your palms facing each other.
2. Press your shoulders back so that your shoulder blades are pushed together.
3. Inhale, raise your shoulders up toward your ears, and let your head drop back.
4. Straighten your arms and lift them away from your buttocks.
5. Exhale, and come to the resting position, as in No. 1.
6. Repeat steps 2, 3, 4, 5 five times. Work up to repeating the exercise for one minute.
7. Let go of your arms and relax. Lightly shake your shoulders. Remind yourself to breathe slightly deeper than you usually breathe throughout the day.

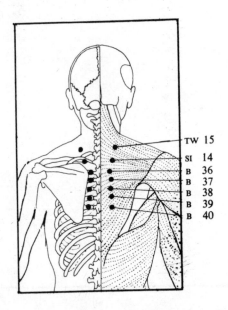

Acu Points	Traditional Associations
Bladder 36, 37	Shoulder spasm or pain, bronchitis, brachial neuralgia, lungs weak, weary and paralyzed.
Bladder 38, 39, 40	Asthma, all types of cardiac disease, slight fever, spasms in the upper back.
Small Intestine 14	Muscular pain and neuralgia of the shoulder and arm, a sensation of coldness circling the shoulder, pneumonia.
Triple Warmer 15	Chest troubled and melancholic, shoulder and back painful, arm and elbow pain when moved.

Benefits: improves poor resistance to illness, upper back and shoulder tensions, cardiac problems, difficult breathing.

Indigestion

Many conditions, including the availability of the various rich and processed foods prevalent in modern life, contribute to the widespread problem of indigestion. Notice how many commercials and advertisements there are for digestive "remedies," and how many people complain of *"foods that don't agree with me."*

This section will cover what can cause indigestion and gas, some considerations for changes you can make in your diet and your eating habits that can improve digestion, and finally some comments on finding what is the right diet for you.

Causes of Indigestion

1. Eating processed, chemically-treated, "devitalized foods" such as artificially colored and preserved meats, dairy products, fruits, and vegetables, and products made with white flour or white sugar or both.
2. Eating heavy or fancy foods such as fried foods, rich sauces, or desserts, which are often difficult to digest.
3. Overeating.
4. Eating foods in improper combinations.
5. Abdominal tension.
6. Lack of exercise.
7. Emotional stress or upset.

Most people are aware of the problems associated with eating processed or overly rich foods, so we will discuss only the other factors that cause digestive problems.

Overeating

Overeating puts a burden on the digestive system. When we eat too much food we overload our digestive organs so that they cannot function properly to fully digest all that we eat. This problem is compounded if what we are eating can cause digestive problems even in regular amounts, such as heavy and rich foods. Rich foods which contain salt or sugar are often consumed in excess because of their addictive qualities.

Overeating can easily cause gas, a product of incompletely digested foods. Eating too much of foods that are rich in fats and oils, such as nuts or fried foods, can especially have this effect.

People overeat for a variety of reasons. Emotional stresses, in particular, can drive someone to overeat. Social pressures, such as overly large portions served at dinner parties or in restaurants, also contribute to problems of overeating. Additionally, overeating is often caused by rushing, or by not paying attention to what you're eating. By chewing thoroughly, and by not distracting yourself when you're eating (by reading, watching TV, etc.) you can eat less and still feel satisfied. Since most of us have a lot of bad habits about eating, it isn't always easy to change, but if you try some of the suggestions made throughout this section, you'll find that the results are worth the effort.

Food Combining

Principles of food combining are based on the fact that certain foods are digested differently than others, so that when they are eaten together neither one can be digested properly. Various foods require both different enzymes and different amounts of time to be digested thoroughly. When eaten together they ferment, causing putrefaction in the digestive system.

It is best to void eating foods from these categories at the same time:
- Fruits with other foods (proteins, starches, vegetables)
- Melons with other foods (including other fruits)
- Different sources of proteins together (nuts, legumes, dairy products, meats)
- Proteins and starches

Good combinations are:
- Fruits with other fruits (except melons)
- Proteins with vegetables
- Starches with vegetables

Experiment with eating foods in proper combinations—you may be surprised with the results!

Abdominal Tension

The digestive organs are located in the abdominal area. Thus, digestion is affected by tension in the abdominal muscles and in the diaphragm, the muscle which separates the thoracic and abdominal cavities. When the digestive organs are subject to excess stress and tensions, their functioning can be hampered, causing indigestion.

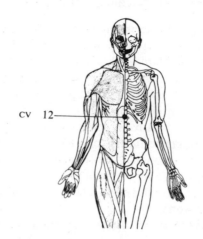

cv 12

Tension in the abdominal muscles, in the diaphragm, or in the digestive organs themselves affects the digestion no matter what, how, or how much you eat. Eventually, when enough tension builds up in the area the digestive process can be impaired. Indigestion, belching, or gas can be the result.

Abdominal tensions can produce a deep irritation in the pit of the stomach. This sometimes unconsciously drives a person to overeat, in an attempt to relieve that tension. In this case an Acupressure point located in this area (Conception Vessel 12, between the navel and the base of the sternum) can be helpful in relieving the irritation. Gradually press into the pit of the stomach at a 45 degree angle towards the diaphragm. Through prolonged pressure on the lump lodged inside this abdominal point, blockages can be broken up and gas expelled.

When your abdominal muscles are relaxed and balanced, the stomach and intestines—which are muscles themselves—are free to work properly. As we breathe fully, the rhythmic movements made by the diaphragm internally massage the stomach. The abdomen needs to be firm (strong, not flabby), with good muscle tone, but also flexible (relaxed, not hard or rigid) to enable the digestive organs to function harmoniously.

Abdominal tensions can be released by practicing the "Bow Pose" given later in this section, and also by the exercise given in the section on *Body Tension*.

Lack of Exercise

Food is the fuel that generates energy for our body; exercise burns up this fuel. Thus, there is a direct link between what you eat and how much exercise you do. Exercise improves circulation, provides an outlet for physical, emotional, and mental tensions, and generally strengthens and tones all the body's muscles. *All* these aspects help improve digestion.

When you exercise regularly, you also tend to develop a healthy appetite, instead of eating from habit, or by a schedule. The tendency to overeat will decrease if you put your body to work. Exercise naturally regulates appetite. When you don't exercise, your metabolism can become sluggish. Improved digestion, assimilation, and elimination are just some of the many benefits of daily exercise.

Emotional and Psychological Aspects

According to Yogic principles, the abdominal area governs the way in which a person deals with his or her personal power. The Solar Plexus nerves in the upper abdomen are directly related to the Third Chakra*, which regulates personal power.

Due to self-doubt, a lack of self-confidence, or fear, people often avoid fully tuning into this part of themselves. Some people accomplish this by overeating, which does release abdominal tension temporarily by creating internal pressures. This, however, further imbalances the digestive system, and does nothing to deal with the emotional cause, which remains to create further problems.

Everyday emotional stresses and tension can also cause indigestion. If you eat when you're upset, it's very difficult to properly digest what you eat. An argument or heated discussion can have this effect, and so can emotions other than anger, such as grief, fear, sadness, and worry.

It's easy to see the direct effect emotional tension and upset can have on the abdomen when you think of common phrases such as *"feeling like I have a knot in my stomach,"* or *"feeling as if I was punched in the gut."* Our "gut level feelings" often refer precisely to the stress in our "guts," that is, our abdomens.

Therefore, whenever possible avoid arguing or getting in an upsetting conversation while you eat. Also avoid eating when you're already emotionally involved in some issue. One technique also found in the "suggestions" part of this section is to take a few moments before you begin to eat and take a few deep breaths. This helps relax and calm you, so that you are in a receptive mood, and not in one that may cause digestive problems.

Gas

One form of indigestion is gas, which can be caused by any of the seven factors listed or discussed above. Gas indicates that food is not being digested completely.

Tension and anxiety can cause gas by creating a tendency to swallow air along with the food. Gas can also be the result of reading or doing something else while eating, or of incomplete chewing of food.

Legumes (beans) are particularly known to cause gas. If beans are cooked properly, however, and eaten in moderation, then gas will not occur. Beans should be soaked in *plain water* for 6–12 hours before cooking. They should also be cooked in plain water. *Do not add salt* until the last 15 minutes of cooking time, when you are seasoning the dish, because cooking beans in salted water will cause gas.

Also, after cooking beans for about 1/2 hour, skim off the blackish foam residue that comes to the top, as this can also cause gas. Cooking beans in this way, and limiting your intake to small portions will enable you to digest beans properly and help avoid gas.

The Right Diet

There are as many dietary options as there are foods on the commercial market, and

---

* See the Chapter on "Chakras" for a further discussion.

there is a spectrum of opinions on the right way to eat. But we are all individuals, and have differing nutritional needs.

The past and present course of our life influences our dietary needs. Every person has a unique combination of past eating habits, parental influences, tastes, lifestyles, physical activity, climate, and metabolism. This great diversity is matched by the diversity of dietary desires and requirements for each individual's optimum health.

The best way to know what is the right diet for you is to experiment with and inform yourself about a variety of ways of eating. *Experience for yourself* what affects different diet have on how you feel. Try different foods, quantities, combinations, ratios. This way you can learn what diet makes you feel best. Remember, however, that it can change! As the seasons change, our dietary needs change also. Gradually change your diet. Extreme changes cause imbalances; therefore, remember to use moderation. It takes a while to gain the benefits of changing your diet. It doesn't happen overnight, although you may experience some immediate results. Be patient and give your body time to adjust.

Suggestions about Eating

● **Relaxation** before and during eating promotes good digestion. The "Prayer Pose Meditation" on page 33 has a balancing and calming effect that promotes harmony. Also, several long, deep breaths before eating helps to relax you, and create a receptive mood in which to enjoy your meal.

● **Give Thanks** to life for the earth, all the natural processes and human efforts that went into creating and cultivating the food you are about to eat, transform, and become.

● **Eat Slowly—Chew Completely**. *This cannot be overemphasized!* Hurried eating and incomplete chewing contributes to indigestion in a number of ways:

(1)   They can indicate an imblanced emotional state of tension, anxiety, and rushing. This almost provides a guarantee of some degree of indigestion. If you only have a small amount of time in which to eat, eat only a small amount of food, and chew it slowly and completely.

(2)   Incomplete chewing hinders digestion because the enzymes in the saliva that begin the digestion process while the food is being chewed don't get a chance to do their job. This puts an added burden on the stomach.

(3)   When you eat quickly you often overeat because you don't give your system the opportunity to signal that it's full. And when you do notice that you're full you're often noticing that you're stuffed! Many people don't stop eating sometimes until they get so full that they have to stop.

(4)   Hurried eating means that you aren't really tasting whatever it is you're gobbling down, and so you aren't even getting the satisfaction you could out of eating.

Deep breathing and thorough chewing will enhance the taste of food and will probably enable you to eat less but get more satisfaction out of what you eat.

● **Drinking While Eating:** Liquids may dilute the essential enzymes necessary to properly digest foods, especially raw or uncooked foods. Generally it is best to drink at least 30 minutes before or after a meal. Drinks that are ice cold can temporarily paralyze the stomach. A little herb tea or a bowl of soup with a meat will probably not hamper digestion.

Acu-Yoga Digestive Aids

The traditional Zen meditation posture of kneeling with your buttocks resting on your heels ("Seiza") promotes good digestion. In this position, various Acupressure points on the tops of the feet are pressed. The digestive organs whose meridians go through this area are the Stomach, Spleen-Pancreas, Liver, and Gall Bladder. Stomach 42, the overall balancing or "source" point of the Stomach Meridian is especially stimulated in "Seiza." Sitting in this position for a few minutes after eating a large meal will improve your digestion.

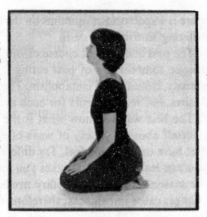

Massaging and gently pressing points around your abdomen (on an empty stomach) can also help to release blockages, tension, and gas in the abdomen. This will increase your awareness of how much tension you have in your abdominal area. It's one way to check the effect of different diets—when your digestion is improved, the soreness and stagnation in your abdomen will begin to lessen.

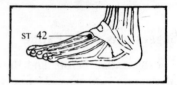

Many of the wise sages in China chose to live in the upper foothills of the mountains. The magnificent beauty of the land and the crisp, sparkling air, away from the hectic pace of cities are possible reasons for their choice of locale. But, they were also aware of the great benefits of walking up steep hills: it flexes the foot in all directions, which stimulates the points and meridians of the feet and ankles. It affects the source points of all the digestive organ meridians, strengthening and balancing them. The next time you walk up a steep hill, remember that you're getting extra benefits for your digestion!

This section, "Indigestion," includes two Acu-Yoga exercises, both of which work on strengthening the entire digestive process. The first one, "Bow Pose," also affects many other aspects of the body. The second, "Wind-Relieving Pose," accomplishes what its name suggests: it helps digestive problems associated with gas.

Bow Pose is one of the most powerful postures for increasing the overall energy of the body and releasing body tension. It has many beneficial effects. It tones the abdominal muscles, helping to reduce abdominal fatness and flabbiness.

As a tonic for the whole body, it strengthens the nervous system, improving brain activity. People who want to improve comprehension and clarity of thought can benefit by regular practice.

Bow Pose is said to affect most of the endocrine glands. It stimulates the thyroid, thymus, liver, kidneys, spleen, pancreas, and sexual glands. Both men and women with characteristic signs of sexual weakness can be helped by daily practice.

Bow Pose effectively releases blockages in the abdominal area by directly pressing central Acupressure points near the stomach. Thus, it has been traditionally used for constipation.

If you wish, you can gently rock back and forth in Bow Pose, inhaling as you go back, and exhaling forward. Be sure to relax immediately after doing the pose for a period of time three times as long as the time you spent in the pose. This will enable you to obtain the greatest benefits of energy circulation. Relaxing deeply after Bow Pose is essential to its effectiveness.

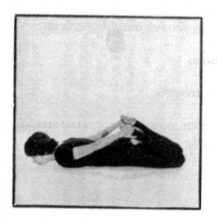 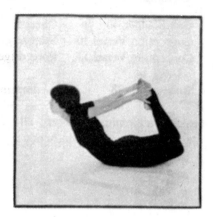

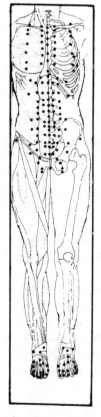

Bow Pose

1. Lie on the stomach. Bring your feet up, bending your knees.
2. Reach back and firmly grasp your feet.
3. Inhale arching the back and bring the head up by pulling on the ankles like a bow.
4. Breathe long and deep through the nose for 20 to 30 seconds. By making the exhalation complete, the internal organs get massaged.
5. Completely allow yourself to relax for a few minutes with your hands facing up, head on its side.

Bow Pose stimulates a series of points on the Governing (GV) and Conception Vessels (CV) and on the Stomach (St) Meridian.

Acu Points	Traditional Associations
Spleen 4	Intestine swollen or painful.
Stomach 42	Balances the Stomach Meridian.
Governing Vessel 4	"Gate of Life"—used in Taoist meditations for energy circulation.
Gall Bladder 40	Chest and ribs painful, breathing difficult.
Conception Vessel 10	Stomachache.
Conception Vessel 11, Liver 14	Poor digestion.
Stomach 21–28	Abdominal problems.

Benefits: abdominal tensions, all digestion organs, the central nervous system, sexual vitality, constipation, cold hands and feet.

Knee Squeeze (Wind Relieving Pose)

The second digestive exercise, Wind-Relieving Pose, helps open up the rectum to expel gas. It also pressed the Acupressure points Stomach 36 and Large Intestine 11, which are strong points that work to improve overall digestion.

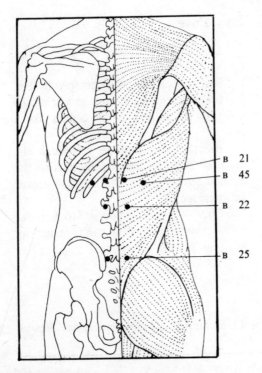

B 21
B 45
B 22
B 25

1. Lie on the back. Comfortably tilt your head back.
2. Bring the knees up to the chest, using your hands to hold Spleen 9 (Sp 9), on the inside of the leg. just underneath the knee bone.
3. Use your arm muscles to help bring your knees to your chest during the exhalation.
4. Inhale. letting the knees come out away from the chest.
5. Enjoy this movement for two minutes.
6. Breathe into the lower abdomen and out of the rectum. Feel the lower back relax and the rectum open with each breath.

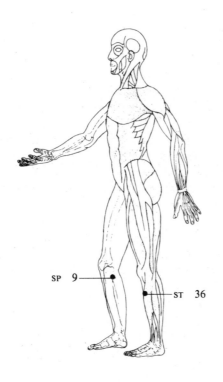

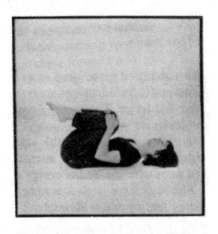

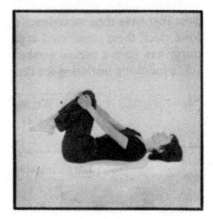

SP 9

ST 36

Acu Points	Traditional Associations
Spleen 9	Knee pains; abdomen heavy.
Stomach 36	Indigestion; abdominal pain or swelling.
Bladder 45	Abdomen distended.
Bladder 21	Stomachache, indigestion.
Bladder 22	Bowels congealed, abdominal pain.
Bladder 25	Constipation, intestinal gas.

Benefits: lower back pain, ache, or stiffness; sciatica, fatigue, constipation, poor digestion, urinary disorders, groaning, belching, snoring, complaining, overeating.

Insomnia

The inability to get to sleep or to stay asleep is often caused by stress and anxiety. Emotional and mental tensions are internalized so that a person is "keyed up" and can't fully relax and let go. The energy flows are imbalanced as a result of the inner pressures and tensions.

Traditional Oriental health care practices say that insomnia is caused by an uneven distribution of energy. The internal blockages cause some meridians to become excessive and some deficient, so the energy cannot flow freely and easily throughout the body.

Although there is always some Ki in every meridian, there is a wave or crest of Ki energy that circulates throughout the meridians of the entire body once every 24 hours. Since there are 12 organ meridians, this means that each meridian is in ascendance for a certain two hour period each day. If the organs that are blocked or excessive in energy are those that have their ascendance during the night, insomnia can result. When the bodily flows reach these constricted organs, their flow is restricted. This condition of blocked energy can keep a person awake.

The following meridians are the ones that are in ascendance late at night:

Triple Warmer	9–11 P.M.
Gall Bladder	11 P.M.–1 A.M.
Liver	1–3 A.M.
Lung	3–5 A.M.
Large Intestine	5–7 A.M.

For example, if a person feels energetic, inspired, or "keyed up," and cannot get to sleep between 11 P.M. and 1 A.M., it may indicate that the Gall Bladder Meridian is excessive. These people tend to work best late at night because they have a surge of energy at this time.

If a person usually wakes up during the night, at about the same time, it can be related to the associated meridian. For example, if a preson has a tendency to eat a lot of oily foods or foods high in cholesterol such as butter and fried foods, their Liver Meridian may become blocked, and they may have trouble sleeping around 1–3 A.M. People with lung problems may wake up between 3–5 A.M.

Becoming aware of one's patterns and feelings according to what time of day or night, it can give you insights into what meridians are blocked. You can then choose an exercise to work on that imbalance. Remember that plenty of outdoor exercise is beneficial for all these meridians. It also helps work out tensions that contribute to insomnia, and results in a physical tiredness that is conductive to good sleep.

According to Chinese Acupuncture, insomnia is also related to the Heart Meridian, so that if a person has an excess amount of energy in that meridian they will have difficulty sleeping. Traditionally, the point, Heart 7* (located on the inside of the wrist, just below the little finger) was used for insomnia. Called "Spirits' Door," this point helps to balance and calm the heart, alleviate anxiety, and enable a person to sleep at night.

---

* Please refer to the drawing on page 192 for the location of this point.

Because of this association with the heart, a diet that places stress on the heart can contribute to insomnia. For example, foods which contain animal fats and chol :rol can block the blood vessels by laying down fatty deposits on their walls. A heart that is forced to overwork and to pump the blood harder through a narrowing vessel can affect one's ability to sleep at night. Salt also has a binding affect on the blood vessels. Therefore, the Chinese traditionally avoided an excessive intake of meat and salt. Limiting your salt intake, substituting granulated dulse, kelp, or a vegetable-herb seasoning, can thus benefit sleep difficulties. Also, some insomnia conditions are caused by blockages in the colon.*

Another cause of insomnia is lack of either social or physical activity. For some people insomnia stems from repressed or blocked motivation, apathy, inactivity, sexual frustration, a lack of personal contact with others, etc. Emotional frustrations "key people up" so they cannot sleep. Also, if you don't use your body enough to feel the healthy fatigue that comes at the end of a full day, you can be restless and not physically tired enough to need rest or be able to rest.

The Acupressure points on the heel have traditionally been used for insomnia. A point on the inside of the heel is called "Joyful Sleep," and one on the outside of the heel is called "Calm Sleep." Massaging and pressing the points on both sides of the heel and the Achilles tendon enable the body to relax and benefit insomnia problems.

Natural Ways to Induce Sleep

 • **Stretch** and induce a few yawns. Feel the tiredness that is often there, but covered up with nervous tension.

 • **Eye problems** exercises, on page 157, starting can help to relieve eyestrain.

 • **Write your own script**, play with your imagination: Make yourself cozy in bed with your eyes closed. Take a few long deep breaths. Picture the things you experienced during the day and accept the day, and whatever it included. Let it flow past. Love yourself for whatever you did and for what you went through today.

 Take three more deep breaths. Picture what tomorrow will be like. Think of what you want to do and how you want to do it. The clearer your projection of that image, the easier it will be to manifest itself tomorrow. Let your mind expand to explore possibilities, things you enjoy. Let yourself relax.

 • **Conscious relaxation exercise:** Lie on your back with your eyes closed. Starting with your toes, tell each part of your body to relax. Go up your entire body; gently move each limb, joint, or muscle to check it out. Let each part of your body relax, one by one.

This exercise, the "Camel Pose," connects points on the Great Bridge Channel, one of the Regulatory Channels which balance energy in the body. Of course, all stretching and relaxation exercises are good for insomnia. "Camel Pose" is especially beneficial because it uses the Acupressure points around the ankles which are traditionally used to calm and deepen sleep.

---

* See the section on "Constipation" for a further discussion of this condition.

Camel Pose

1. Sit on your heels, and then open your legs so that you are between them.
2. Reach back and grab your ankles. Inhale, arching your back and buttocks up, holding your heels.
3. Breathe long and deeply in this position for 30 seconds.
4. Slowly come down. Place your thumbs on Bladder 2 (the inside upper ridge of the eye socket bone) and bend forward, resting on the ground for two minutes.

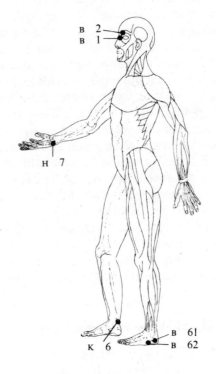

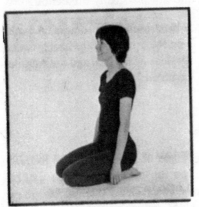

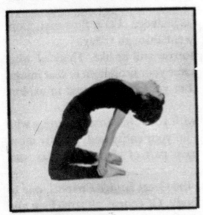

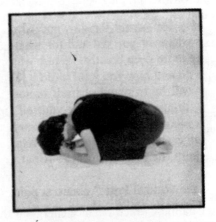

Acu Points	Traditional Associations
Kidney 6	Stage fright, madness at night, insomnia.
Bladder 61, 62	"Calm Sleep," insomnia, tension headache.
Bladder 1, 2	Eye tensions, headache, brain tired.

Benefits: the bladder and kidneys, chills, nervous conditions, fatigue.

Menstrual Tension

There are both physical and emotional causes of menstrual cramps. As with all symptoms, menstrual tension and cramps are a signal of an imbalance in the body.

Physical Conditions

Problems associated with cramps are pelvic tension or congestion, uterine inflammation or swelling, constipation, a contracted cervix, and hormone imbalances, including weakness or imbalance of the thyroid and parathyroid glands and the ovaries. These glands secrete hormones that regulate menstruation and metabolism. Doctors commonly prescribe estrogen or progesterone hormones to treat menstrual irregularities. Constant practice of Acu-Yoga over a period of time, however, can naturally stimulate the endocrine system to regulate these hormones. The results from natural methods take longer but they do not have the side effects of synthetic drugs.

Emotional Conditions

Menstrual problems can also have emotional roots, since the emotional state greatly influences the hormonal balance. Fear, worry, anger and irritation can thus create stress, tensions and imbalances which contribute to menstrual cramps.

Changes of weather or locale can also affect our emotions and our hormonal balance.

"Such conditions influence the interbrain which governs emotional reactions, ovulation, and the secretion of hormones from the anterior lobe of the pituitary gland."[36]

Prevention

Prior to and during menstruation, women, especially those who have menstrual problems, generally need rest, warmth, moderate exercise, and a nurturing environment. Women have a great capacity to nurture others; the duration of her period is a good time for a woman to take care of herself. Warm blankets and clothing, avoidance of stressful situations, rest, and making time for personal interests are all examples of conditions that create a supportive environment.

With regards to diet, calcium is one of the most important minerals for preventing menstrual cramps. It enables the nerves and muscles to relax. Calcium levels drop substantially during the week before menstruation; low levels of calcium can cause pre-menstrual tension, bloating, and nervous headaches.

There are many foods that supply the body with calcium, and can thus help prevent cramps if eaten during the week before menstruation. Fresh green leafy vegetables such as

---

[36] Katsusuki Serizawa, M.D., *Massage: The Oriental Method*, page 68.

lettuce, spinach, kale, parsley (which can be steeped for tea), collards, and turnip greens are naturally high in calcium. Magnesium is also important, since it complements the absorption of calcium. Sea vegetables, seeds, and nuts contain high amounts of both of these minerals.

Tofu, a traditional high-protein food made from soy beans, can be prepared with a little fresh grated ginger and served with green vegetables for assimilation of calcium and iron. Asparagus in the spring, strawberries in the summer, cucumbers in the fall, and parsnips in the winter are foods which also contain these valuable nutrients. Dairy products also contain calcium.

Cranberry juice and sasparilla root are natural diuretics which help bloating and water retention problems. Red raspberry leaves decrease the menstrual flow (without stopping it) to ease menstrual tension.

Women often have lower back and abdominal tension during menstruation. Regular practice of Acu-Yoga to strengthen and release tension in these areas can also help reduce menstrual discomfort.

Alternative Self-Treatments for Releasing Menstrual Tension

- Apply a hot water bottle, heating pad, or hot towel to the small of the back. Cover the body with a blanket.
- Apply a light mustard plaster to the abdomen. Mix one part ground mustard seed with five parts whole wheat flour. Mix with warm water to make a paste thick enough to spread on a piece of cheesecloth. Then place the cheesecloth over the lower abdomen. Leave on until it fully warms the abdomen. After removing the mustard plaster, lie down and cover yourself with a warm blanket.
- Do the "Meditation for Exploring the Cause of Disease" on page 44 to discover the cause of your discomfort. Open your mind to receive the messages contained in your cramps. A common tendency is to avoid both the pain and the reason behind it. Challenge yourself to go beyond superficial treatment of a symptom to the underlying roots of the condition.
- Hot or cold application can release menstrual tension. Heat from saunas or baths increases the menstrual flow; cold decreases the flow. If your flow is heavy to begin with, heat is not appropriate. In any case, it is best to avoid extremes.

A few years ago a friend of mine had what seemed to be severe menstrual cramps. Although it was only 21 days since her last period, she had such pain in her lower abdomen that I almost felt she needed emergency medical attention. We had planned to go out for the evening, but since that was out of the question, we decided to stay home. Before picking her up, I did some research, and found out that ginger tea was traditionally used in both China and India for menstrual cramps. I made a tea of fresh, chopped ginger root, simmered in several cups of water for 20 minutes. (If you try this, use a stainless steel, glass, or enamel pot—avoid aluminum.) She and I both consumed two large mugfulls of this tea as we talked. Afterwards I began giving her an Acupressure session. In the middle of the session, she had to get up to go to the bathroom. Her cramps had somewhat subsided but she still felt some pain. After 10 minutes, however, she came out of the bathroom, her face flushed, beaming with a wonderful smile. "My period," she said with relief, "it came, just now, and I feel great."

The following Acu-Yoga exercise, "Pelvic Stretch," stimulates points traditionally associated with menstrual cramps. The techniques contained in the section on "Pelvic Tension" are also excellent for releasing and preventing menstrual cramps.

Pelvic Stretch

1. Lie on your back.
2. Bend your knees, spreading your feet apart, placing them flat on the floor.
3. Grab ahold of your ankles, palms on the outside and fingers on the inside, holding your inside shin three fingers' width above the ankle bone.
4. Inhale and arch the pelvis up.
5. Exhale and relax the pelvis down.
6. Continue for one minute, inhaling up and exhaling down.

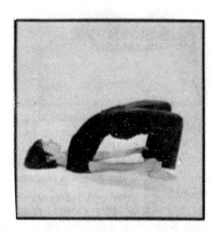

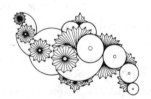

Relaxation: To Enhance the Release of Menstrual Tension

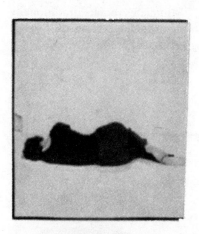

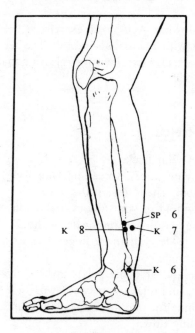

1. Curl up on your side in fetus position.
2. Interlock the large and second toes of one foot onto the Achilles tendon area of the other.
3. With your eyes closed, gently rock your body back and forth for a few minutes, stimulating the points on either side of the heel. The Acupressure points in the hips that are beneficial for menstrual cramps will be pressed in this position.

4. Roll over on your other side, repeating steps No. 1, 2, and 3 with the opposite foot. Close your eyes and nurture yourself as you rock for another few minutes.
5. Turn over on your back and completely relax.

Acu Points	Traditional Associations
Spleen 6	Pressure or pain in the genitalia of both sexes, abdomen swollen, insomnia, menstrual cramps, nervous depression.
Kidney 6 "Bigger Stream"	Irregular periods, sores on both legs, heel swollen and painful, impotence.
Kidney 7 "Returning Current"	Abdomen distended like a drum, limbs swollen, edema, constipation, fatigue, back pains, cannot bear to move.
Kidney 8 "Exchange Letters"	Menstruation irregularity, red and white discharge, prolapse of the uterus, loins, thighs, and legs painful, abdominal pain on one side.

Benefits: the spleen, liver, and kidneys, sexual frustrations, pelvic tensions, the uterus, impotency, diarrhea, insomnia, cold feet.

Neck Tension

The Chinese have called the neck the "pillar of heaven" because in a healthy, relaxed person the mind is calm and at peace. The neck, however, is also the *first area* of the body where tension hits. Therefore, whenever a person is under any sort of stress—whether from personal, social, or work demands—the neck is one area that always becomes tense.

The Fight or Flight Reflex

This is part of an ancient reflex, from the time when stress meant physical danger and tensing the neck area helped protect the head and the exposed blood vessels on the throat. Although most stress today is caused by situations that don't require a physical response, the old patterns still function. Thus, whether the stressful situation is primarily physical, mental, or emotional, we still respond by unconsciously tightening the neck muscles.

Further, the feelings that go along with these pressures and demands of everyday life often remain unexpressed, resulting in corresponding emotional tensions. These blocked feelings, and other unfinished emotional business, are also stored in the neck.

Since many people either do not know how to relieve this stress, or don't practice the techniques that they do know, the tensions build and can become chronic. Neck tension, pain, stiffness, and even pinched nerves in the neck are therefore, unfortunately, very common.

Whenever the neck is strained for any reason, it becomes difficult for it to properly fulfill its responsibility of supporting the weight of the head, which is usually 15 to 20 pounds. Stresses and strains create an additional burden on the neck muscles, and an unhealthy situation is set up where tension breeds more tension.

The Neck and the Meridians

Another factor involved in neck tension is that many of the meridians travel through the neck, which is a small area. Therefore, when there is tension in the neck, these flows can intermingle and cause complications, such as stiffness, sore throat, or swollen glands.

The Acupressure points in the neck area are known as "windows of the sky" (see chart at end of this section). When the neck is strong, flexible, and in proper alignment, these "windows" are clear and open—that is, we are open to the flow of life, and experience its harmonious nature. When tension interferes, however, it can affect us on all levels, and we become more closed physically, emotionally, mentally, and spiritually. Since the neck is such a key area, and so prone to build-ups of tension, it is especially important to practice techniques to unblock it.

Physical Tensions

Some neck tensions are caused by problems that are mainly physical. Hard physical labor, for example, can often strain the neck. Also, certain jobs directly create neck tension by requiring that the neck be held in an awkward position for long periods of time.

Mental Tensions

Mental tensions can also affect the neck. People who strain themselves mentally by excessive thinking and planning are all too familiar with the fatigue and tension in the neck area that are caused by these efforts. Our culture tends to emphasize the intellectual, and neglect the physical and emotional aspects of life, so that we are especially prone to the mental stresses that cause neck problems.

Emotional Tensions

Neck tension can also be caused by emotional imbalances. When we tense our bodies in response to anger, fear, or frustration, the neck is affected. Over a period of time there can be a great accumulation of tenseness and stiffness in the neck area. In fact, often this is created by tensing *against* our emotions, that is, unconsciously tightening the muscles in an attempt to block out the pain and frustration in our lives. Unfortunately, the more we repress our emotions, the more we armor ourselves muscularly, and the worse the tension gets. One very blatant example of the extent to which neck tension is a part of our culture is the widespread use of the common phrase, "a pain in the neck" to describe a person or situation in response to which one feels frustration or anger.

The following diagram illustrates the association between segments of neck tension, the meridians, and emotions.

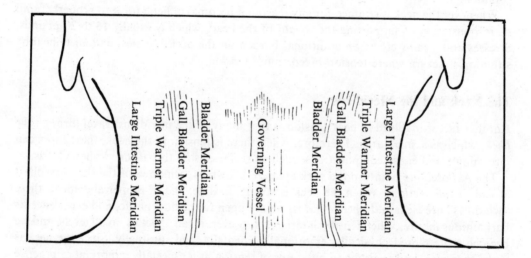

Emotion	Organ meridian	Hypofunction	Hyperfunction
anger	Liver/Gall Bladder	indecisive	irritation
fear	Bladder/Kidneys	doubt	foolhardiness
grief	Large Intestines/Lungs	sorrow	holding
joy	Triple Warmer/Pericardium	confusion	distress

Self-Expression

The neck is a barometer for self-expression. The expression of our feelings, thoughts, hopes, and plans is a basic need for all people. Since self-expression relates to the Fifth Chakra, which is located at the base of the throat, blocked expression can directly affect the neck, causing stagnation and tension.

If we express ourselves appropriately—at a proper time, in a proper place, and in a proper way—we can maintain a harmonious balance within ourselves, and between ourselves and the world, and probably keep ourselves free of neck tension. While we are still in the process of unfolding, and learning to master the art of harmonizing with the changes of the flow of life, however, we probably will have some neck tension!

Mind and Body Interactions

The neck registers the interaction between the dictates of the mind and the needs of the body. Neck tension, therefore, accumulates when the mind and body are in conflict, or when the needs of one are neglected because of the other's demand. For instance, if your body needs to relax because it is tired, but your mind is telling you that you should work, then there is conflict. Conversely, if your body needs activity but your mind says you should "go home to relax," there is also conflict. This dissension usually registers in the neck.

A disharmony between the mind and body is also often created when the issue of sexual activity arises. Sometimes your body is too tense or tired to feel receptive to love-making, but your mind may have expectations about having a sexual experience. On the other hand, your body may feel aroused and want to "neck" while your mind is telling you for some reason that you shouldn't.

Towards Harmonious Living

When mind and body are in harmony with each other, when work is balanced with play, when one's life has a harmonious rhythm, then the neck remains flexible and agile. "*Regularity in habit, in action, in repose, in eating, in drinking, in sitting, in walking, in everything, gives one that rhythm which is necessary and which completes the music of life.*"[37]

Pillar of Heaven Pose

1. Kneel on the floor and sit on your heels.
2. Inhale, and clasp your hands together behind your neck. Lean forward as you exhale, and place your head on the floor. Tuck the chin into the chest.
3. Raise your buttocks up and gently move forward on the top of your head, stretching the neck muscles. Breathe long and deep.
4. Slowly turn your head a little to each side and gently lean forward so that other areas of the neck are stretched. The sore points on the top of the head facilitate the

---

[37] Sufi Inayat Khan, *The Book of Health*, page 6.

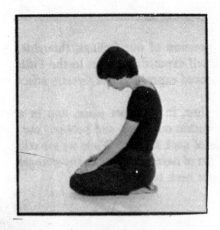 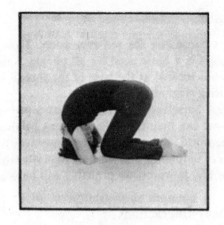

release of chronic neck tensions.

a minute.

5. Continue to stretch the neck, for about

6. Relax for a few minutes on your back.

Windows of the Sky Pose

1. Lie on your back. Clasp your hands together behind your neck.

2. Exhale, and slowly pull the head up, using your arm muscles. The heels of the palms should be firmly pressing the sides of your neck.

3. Do *Hara* breathing*, keeping the head up in this manner. Eyes are closed. Relax into the pose for one minute.

4. Bring the elbows together, stretching further.

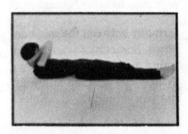

5. Inhale and slowly lower the head to the floor. Relax with your arms by your sides and discover the benefits.

Acu Points	Traditional Associations
Stomach 6	Neck rigid, difficult to turn, facial acne.
Governing Vessels 15, 19 and 20.	Head and neck stiff, headaches, insomnia.
Bladder 6 and 7	Head feels heavy, headache (top of the head).
Bladder 8	Rheumatism of the neck and shoulders.
Gall Bladder 12 and 20	Neck painful or stiff.

Benefits: sore throat, acne, stiff neck, thyroid irregularities, congestion or itching in the throat, mental disorders, speech problems, general pain.

* Slow, deep breaths into the lower abdominal region.

200

"The Windows of the Sky"

Name	Point	Location on the neck	Traditional Associations
"Man Welcome"	St 9	Front	Throat swollen red and painful, hypertension, asthma.
"Support and Rush"	LI 18	Front edge	Cough, shortness of breath, sore throat, pain in the opposite hip.
"Heaven Rushing"	CV 22	Front in the center	Dry cough, noise in throat like a bird, sores in throat, swollen throat, congested or stiff tongue.
"Heavenly Window"	SI 16	Side in the middle	Spasm in the neck and shoulder, lethargy, inability to twist the neck due to stiffness.
"Heavenly Appearance"	SI 17	Side under ear lobe	Swelling and immobility of the neck, sore throat, nausea, tonsillitis.
"Window of Heaven"	TW 16	Back edge	Shoulder, back, and arms painful, stiff neck, face swollen, eyes painful.
"Heavenly Pillar"	B 10	Back	Head heavy, spasms in the neck muscles, nose blocked, swollen throat.
"Wind Mansion"	GV 16	Middle of back at base of skull	Headache, stiff neck, fear, deafness, mental disorders, eyes move wildly, suicidal.

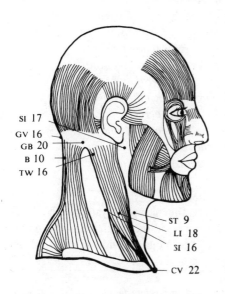

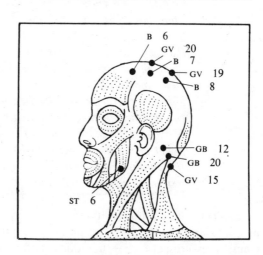

Nervous Disorders

A great many factors contribute to a weakening of the nerves: stress and strain of work and family situations; a sedentary lifestyle which doesn't provide the exercise needed for health; a diet of mainly processed foods, including a lot of salt, sugar, white flour; injuries or accidents; extensive use of cars and airplanes for transportation; poor posture; and spinal misalignment.

The latter is especially important because the body's nerves, which come out to all areas of the body from the spine, can be damaged or "pinched" when the discs between the vertebrae are misaligned or deteriorate*. A combination of the factors listed above contribute to these imbalances in the spine and in the nerves.

Exercise and diet are also important because without enough exercise and healthy food, the body deteriorates. This gradual wearing down is easiest to see in older people, whose bodies have been abused for so long that they have deteriorated sooner and to a greater extent than necessary. Consequently, elderly people are more prone to develop nerve disorders.

Although neurologists have highly developed technological ways to test and diagnose, it is rare to find a doctor who prescribes natural methods for improving the nerves. Typically, braces and traction are used to immobilize the affected parts of the body, and pain killers are used to numb them. This type of treatment may be appropriate for extreme cases of debility, but there is an exciting potential for the use of therapeutic exercises, diet, Acupressure, and massage for improving nerve conditions.

> "*Physicians, especially those who practice in large cities, are often consulted by individuals who, although not manifesting a well-defined disease, are evidently not in good health. It is possible that these cases do not receive as much attention from friends of the person, or even from the physician her/himself, as they deserve, for the tendency . . . is to ignore or make light of the symptoms presented. In nervous exhaustion, moreover, the indications of the difficulty are of a subjective rather than of an objective character, that is, they are symptoms which the patient can him/herself feel, but which no one else can perceive . . . . Nervous exhaustion is an affliction of modern society, and is found in the most aggravated types in the United States. For the causes that stimulate the mind to excessive exertion are especially active in this country.*"[38]

Acu-Yoga is a powerful therapeutic way of toning the nervous system. The body positions and the Acupressure points strengthen the nerves directly through the movements, pressures, stretches, breathing, and relaxation. Acu-Yoga provides a deep release

---

* Please see "Spinal Disorders" for a discussion of this issue.

[38] Lyman, Fenger, and Belfield, *The New Century Family Physicians Cyclopedia of Medical Reference*, pages 355–356.

of tension that relaxes and revitalizes the entire body. Its emphasis on the spine makes it an ideal practice for developing a strong and balanced nervous system.

Reflexology

According to Yogic teachings, many of the 72,000 nerves of the body have endings in the feet. The soles of the feet are an orderly reflection of the entire body, with head-to-foot related to toe-to-heel. Therefore, a problem in the head area, such as sinus blockages, would show up on the feet in the toe region. Both feet are involved, so that the "middle" of the two feet put together, that is, the arches, represent the spine, which runs down the middle of the body.

Foot massage is therapeutic for many conditions. Pressure on the arches is especially beneficial for nerve disorders. Massage the feet two or three times daily for 10 minutes, or walk barefoot on unpaved ground to massage the feet. We often hold a lot of tensions in our feet, and giving them a little attention feels wonderful!

Dollar Pose

1. Lie on your back with your feet together.
2. Inhale and raise your legs up over your head.
3. Use your hands to hold both sides of your heels.
4. Adjust the angle of your legs by bending your knees to apply pressure between the shoulder blades.
5. Relax in the posture and breathe long and deep for one minute.
6. Completely relax on your back with your eyes closed for a few minutes, feeling your blood and energy circulate.

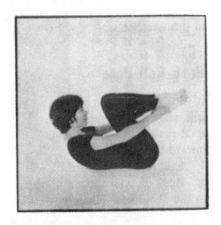

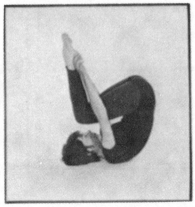

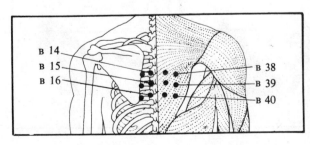

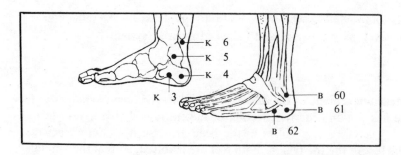

Acu Points	Traditional Associations
Bladder 60, 61, 62	Tension headaches, lumbago, sciatica.
Kidney 3, 4, 5, 6	Insomnia, asthma, constipation, headaches.
Governing Vessel 11, 12	Forgetfulness, nervousness, rigid spine.
Bladder 14, 15, 16, 38, 39, 40	Hypertension, upper back pain, cardiac problems.

Benefits: liver, thyroid and nervous disorders, back pain.

The second exercise for this section, "Rock-Roll Pose," is also good for stiffness in the back, neck, and legs, sciatica, hypertension, and circulation. The Acupressure points on the toes are held, which has an overall balancing effect. The entire back is also loosened in this exercise.

Rock-Roll Pose

1. Lie on a padded surface on your back with your legs togehter.
2. Inhale, raising your arms and legs up toward the sky.
3. Exhale, and grab hold of your toes.
4. Rock on your spine from the buttocks to the shoulders. Inhale as you come up and exhale as you go back; breathe with the movement.
5. Continue for about a minute. Allow your legs to bend as you rock back and forth.
6. Inhale and slowly lower your legs. Relax on your back.

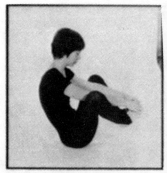
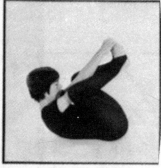
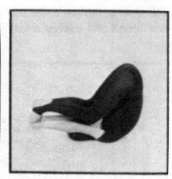

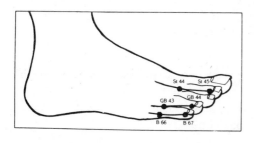

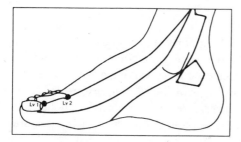

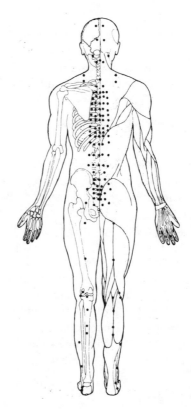

Bladder Meridian and Governing Vessel Points

Acu Points	Traditional Associations
Bladder 11 through 25 Governing Vessels 1 through 14	The spinal nerves that correspond to all of the internal organs. Preventive for fevers, stiff back, hypertension, and nervousness.
Bladder 36 through 49	Rheumatism, backache, kidney weakness, stiffness all over.
Liver 1, 2	Insomnia, gastric pain, lower abdomen swollen, epileptic fits.
Stomach 44, 45	Nightmares, pain with fear and trembling, abdomen distended.
Gall Bladder 43, 44	Nightmares, spasms in the toes, vertigo, rib painful.
Bladder 66, 67	Vertigo, fear, indigestion, gastritis.

Benefits: intercostal neuralgia, edema, influenza, back pains and tension, weariness.

Pelvic Tension

Pelvic tension is a very common condition since the pelvis is an area of the body which is exposed to a great deal of stress, and therefore easily accumulates tension. It is therefore important to practice techniques which help release tension from the pelvis, if you want to improve your strength, flexibility, and overall balance.

Shock Absorber and Hinge

The pelvis connects the upper and lower body and supports the weight of the upper body on the legs. It also acts as a shock absorber for the spine, protecting the spine and upper body from the impact of the body weight, especially during walking and running.

It provides for a great range of body movement, with the overall posture of the body being determined by the position of the pelvis. Therefore, when the pelvis is pulled out of place or stagnated by tension, the whole body is affected. Conversely, if the posture of another part of the body is poor, the pelvis cannot properly do its job of distributing the body weight, and muscle strain and joint tension in the pelvic region can result.

There are many important muscles, tendons, ligaments, nerves, arteries, and lymph nodes in this area. Approximately 36 muscles attach to the pelvis; they act together to stabilize the pelvic girdle in relation to the spine. When all of the muscles, tendons, and so forth work together harmoniously, they contribute to the optimum condition of the body in general. However, because there is so much going on within this one area, it is all too common for there to be blockages, instead of balance.

The Meridians

This situation is compounded by the fact that there are also many meridians which run through the relatively small groin area in the front of the pelvic girdle, namely the Stomach, Spleen, Kidney, and Liver Meridians. In some places these meridians are not only close together, but actually cross over each other. In addition, the Gall Bladder Meridian runs over the side of the pelvic area, and the Bladder Meridian runs through the back. Because of all this activity, tension can accumulate around key Acupressure points of these meridians, especially in the area where the top of the thighbone is inserted into the hip socket of the pelvis. Blockages in the meridians can cause physical problems.

Effects on Pelvic Organs

Tension in the pelvis directly affects the reproductive and digestive organs. When the muscles and meridians of the pelvic area are tense or stagnated the colon can become blocked, and the circulation of both blood and nervous system impulses to the genitals is reduced. For the sexual sensations to be as full as possible, the pelvic area must be flexible.

The following are some of the conditions that can contribute to tension in the pelvis:

Restrictive Clothing: Fashion strongly influences how we carry ourselves, which unfortunately is usually in an unhealthy way. For example, it is fashionable to appear slim, which can result in a lot of pelvic and abdominal tension, as people tighten their stomachs in an attempt to meet the fashion "ideal." Girdles were created for this very purpose. Tight pants and other tapered clothes, which are cut to bring out this slim look, add to the problem. The result is tension, decreased flexibility and mobility of the pelvis, and impaired functioning of the pelvic organs.

Poor Posture and Lack of Movements: The pelvis is designed to move in all directions. A sedentary life style in which sitting at desks, riding in cars, and waiting in lines is a common routine stagnates the body, since it does not have an opportunity to be fully moved and stretched. This lack of movement becomes a permanent pattern, tension builds, and the area becomes more and more tight and congested. Thus, the posture of the entire body is poor, the entire skeletal frame being thrown out of position. This is so common; look around and see how few people have fluid, strong posture, and how many have their knees locked, pelvises protruding backwards (producing a swayback), and shoulders hunched up.

Under the brunt of this bad posture the pelvis becomes rigid, almost locked into one position. This impairs circulation, weakens genital functioning, and can cause constipation, lumbago, sciatica, and impotency. It's easy to see that posture is important.

Chest and Shoulder Tension: There is a direct relationship between tension in upper and lower portions of the spine. When one is out of proper alignment, a strain is put on the other to compensate, so that you end up with tension and poor alignment in both areas. Since most people are more aware of their shoulder tension than their pelvic tension, it is important to work on the pelvis to cultivate an awareness of the tension stored there, and of whatever blocked or stagnated energies are present there. The depth of the breath is also a barometer for pelvic tension. The breathing cannot be full and deep if there is tension in the chest, or abdominal and pelvic areas.

Emotional Association and Frustrations: The pelvis is also considered the gate of the abdomen, where we experience our "gut level" feelings. Abdominal tensions can block off these feelings, so that we tend to lose touch with our true needs and desires. Our emotions and their expressions are inhibited by tensions and repressions. This, of course, results in *frustration*, since no matter what we do, our deep needs remain unmet. Many people are stuck in this frustration, since the substitute "gratifications" they turn to in an attempt to relieve this frustration are destructive habits—such as smoking, drinking, or overeating, and eating non-nutritional foods solely for taste or sensation—which not only does not satisfy the person, but which weaken and toxify the body, making the true satisfaction of health and openness more and more elusive.

The flip side of this negative situation is one where pelvic tensions, and their associated emotions, are gradually released in a balanced way. Releasing pelvic tension can enable a person to liberate him or herself from anxiety, worry, and fear, and to then more fully experience inner gratification, and to move forward in life.

Sexual Repressions

Culturally we are taught to block the sexual feelings of our genitals. The "don't touch—bad boy/girl!" is hardly conductive to a healthy, relaxed pelvis, but parental admonitions needn't be so outspoken to have a powerful inhibiting effect. Difficult or stressful experiences in toilet training can have a similar result. This closing down of the natural mobility and feeling in the pelvic area is accomplished by tightening the muscles of the pelvic region, to dull and deaden sensation, repressing the sexual feelings.

A number of problems, such as impotency, lack of sexual drive, weak erection, premature ejaculation, vaginal infections, and menstrual cramps can eventually result from the imbalances caused by pelvic blockages. Even if the condition does not degenerate to this point, the reproductive organs can still be weakened by pelvic tension. In this case, orgasm often serves as a temporary release of stress.

When tension in the pelvic region is released, it is possible to experience a depth of feeling that was previously impossible; when this area is free, loose, and open, pleasurable sensations can circulate in a deep and satisfying way.

All of these various problems—restrictive clothing, poor posture and lack of movement, chest and shoulder tension, and emotional stresses, especially frustration and sexual repressions—add up to a cultural pattern of pelvic and abdominal tension that hinders the development of us all. It's a key area of blockage that's important to focus on when you're working to balance yourself as a whole.

The following Acu-Yoga pose, "Locust Pose," works on the Acupressure points in this area and can increase the blood supply and sensory impulses to the entire pelvic region. It is an excellent example of the way in which the traditional Yogic postures utilize Acupressure, since pressure is directly put on specific Acupressure points in the groin area. This pose works to unblock muscular tensions in the lower back, groin, genital and abdominal regions. Daily practice can improve posture, elimination, menstrual disorders, potency, and other sexually-related problems.

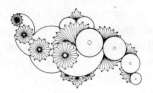

Locust Pose

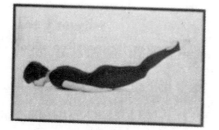

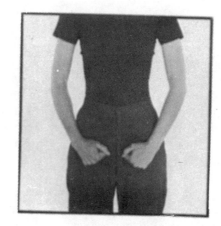

1. Lie down on your stomach with your feet together. Rest your head on either your chin or your forehead.
2. Make your hands into fists, and put them under your hips so that they fit inside the front hip bones near the groin.
3. Inhale deeply, lifting your legs as high as possible, keeping the legs straight and feet together.
4. Keep your legs up and breathe deeply into your *Hara* (lower abdomen) for about 30 seconds.
5. Inhale deeply and raise the legs up further, then hold for 10 seconds.
6. Turn your head to the side and completely relax.

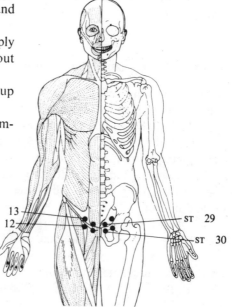

Acu Points	Traditional Associations
Spleen 12	Abdominal pain or swelling.
Spleen 13	Pain in buttocks, hernia, indigestion.
Stomach 29	Genital balancing.
Stomach 30	Sexual potency.

Benefits: the genital and abdominal regions, frustration, groin pains, constipation, digestive problems, cold feet.

Potency

In terms of Chinese physiology, potency depends in general on the overall condition of the human body and in particular on the condition of the kidneys.

The human body is composed of an interconnected network of vital systems united by Ki, or life energy. All functions of the body, including sexuality, depend on the state of this Ki. The body is able to store this human energy (Chen Chi), thus creating reserved energy (Ching Chi). This reserved energy is avilable to be used as needed for various body functions, including sexuality. The Ching Chi, which can be transmuted into sexual energy, is stored in the kidneys; therefore, the condition of the kidneys is directly associated with potency.*

When the kidneys have an abundance of this reserved energy, the functioning of the vital organs is strong and regular. Impotency, on the other hand, resuts from weakness or depletion of kidney energy.

Both daily habits and unusual or stressful situations affect potency. Depending on how we live, how we respond to the circumstances of our life, we can either build or deplete our energy reserves. In this section we will look at the different types of impotency, their causes, and ways of strengthening the reproductive system.

Types of Impotency and Their Causes

There are several types of impotency. *The Ayurveda*, an East Indian classic of medicine, classified impotency under the following main headings:

1. **Emotional:** Emotional imbalances can affect potency, whether they are associated with intimate relationships or with other circumstances of life.

In close relationships, impotency can be due to a lack of mutual emotional responsiveness. The tension and anxiety that can result in the absence of openness and communication between people is worsened by inner pressures of expectations, fears, lack of confidence, and insecurity.

In its highest form, sex is an expression of love, tenderness, and intimacy. When it is done solely for physical sensation and gratification, with no sharing and caring, problems and dissatisfaction are inevitable. When people treat each other as sex objects, lovemaking is reduced to a mutual masturbation which sooner or later becomes unfulfilling. This kind of sexuality fosters anxiety, insecurity, and other negative feelings which then become associated with sex, so that the love, trust and intimacy necessary for a satisfying, long lasting relationship are even less likely to grow.

Pressures to act in certain expected ways develop when sex is based on performance instead of love. Often, men ejaculate prematurely, without conscious control, as an unconscious release of these pressures in the relationship. Or, if men fantasize excessively so that they are already aroused, the semen can accumulate and can be more quickly ejaculated during intercourse. In women, vaginal infections, menstrual cramps, or other problems related to the genitals can be an expression of emotional stress and pressure.

---

* Remember that the term "kidney" in Acu-Yoga refers not only to the physical organ but also to the meridian and points associated with it.

In other aspects of life, dependency and fear are related to the kidneys, and therefore to potency. Impotency can be related to feelings of guilt, self-doubt, fear, or foolhardiness. The more fearful people tend to be, the more clinging or insecure (excess yin) they can become. The other extreme of egocentric, overbearing people (excess yang) tend to be foolhardy and to push themselves beyond their limits in order to prove how unafraid they are. Both extremes can weaken the kidneys and affect potency. Of course, both extremes also cause problems in interpersonal relationships, creating a negative cycle.

2. **Biliary Impotency:** When a person is in a poor state of health, blockages can form in the gall bladder and liver, so that bile accumulates. This has a strong debilitating effect on the nerves, glands, and blood. These blockages inhibit the production and distribution of semen, which can result in an inability to ejaculate. The proper secretion of bile can also be affected by drinking alcohol and taking drugs.

Emotionally, the liver is associated with anger. Repressed anger is common in our culture where strict morals are worshipped. Anger that is pushed down and held inside can also affect the liver, resulting in biliary impotency.

3. **Inappropriate Celibacy:** Abstaining from sex is a traditional Yogic practice. It can be very valuable, but it also can be inappropriate or forced, in which case it can have a negative effect on sexuality and sexual function.

Traditionally, celibacy is one element in a program of physical purification. Like fasting, it can be used as a tool for cleansing the system and for learning about oneself, but the tool can be misused. Fasting, whether from sex or from food, should only be done at the right time and in the right circumstances of one's life. It does no good if it's being done from an external pressure of "should" rather than from an inner feeling that feels right as a form of self-discipline.

4. **Dissipation:** Each individual has his or her own level of sexual need, of balance of sexual activity. Like any activity, sex can be overdone. An excess of sexual activity can dissipate or drain a person's reserve energies, and can eventually result in partial impotency.

5. **Organic Impotency:** A lifestyle that generally deteriorates health can also cause impotency. A number of different habits and conditions can deplete the kidneys, thereby affecting potency. These include eating white sugar, drinking excess fluids, exposure to cold, overall fatigue, and chronic lower back problems.

White sugar is a great enemy of the kidneys. Metabolizing sugar puts a strain on the adrenal glands, which are located directly on top of, and are closely linked with the kidneys.

Excess fluids also tax the kidneys, requiring them to work harder in the process of filtration. This is also true in terms of the Oriental Five Elements Theory, in which the kidneys are associated with the Water Element, so that an excess of that element damages the related organ.

Contrary to Western thinking, a lot of water is detrimental to the kidneys. For proper balance it's best to drink moderate amounts of liquid only. The common practice of supposedly "cleansing" the body by "flushing" it with large amounts of fluids, along with a large consumption of sugar, are cultural causes of impotency.

Cold is another factor that influences the condition of the kidneys. Therefore, whether the cold is in the form of one intense prolonged exposure, or from repeated milder ones, the kidneys and reproductive system can be damaged by it. A lack of warm clothing or bedding during cold weather, especially when endured over a period of time, can cause this type of organic impotency. Similarly, eating cold foods, such as cold drinks or ice cream, especially in the fall and winter, can damage the kidney energy reserves.

In moderation, however, cold can strengthen both the body as a whole, the kidney energy reserve, and the sexual organs. For instance, taking a cold shower for a few minutes each day can build kidney energy.

Fatigue is another element that contributes to organic impotency. Traditionally the winter season is a time to retreat.

> "*As the power of the dark winter ascends, the light retreats to security so that the dark coldness cannot damage one's vitality. This retreat is natural in order to not exhaust one's forces.*"[39]

To be harmoniously balanced with the seasons it's important to cultivate your energy in the spring; build and strengthen it in the summer; gather and store it in the fall; and conserve your energy during the winter months. This is important for maintaining health and is essential for developing potency. Without a seasonal perspective, fatigue can drain away the body's natural energy reserves.

The lower back and the kidneys are directly interrelated. The kidneys are physically located in the lower back. A portion of the Kidney Meridian and special kidney Acupressure points can also be found there. Therefore, if someone's lower back area is stiff or weak, the kidneys can be affected. Since many people have lower back problems, it's important to exercise and stretch this area. Because of the link between the kidneys and potency, people who have lower back problems may also have sexual or reproductive difficulties.

Basically, by not taking care of yourself you can deplete the strength of your vital organs, resulting in organic impotency. Depending upon the length of time, the extent of unhealthful habits, and the strength of one's original constitution, this type of impotency can be corrected by developing your potency as discussed below.

5. **Genital Infections:** Syphilis or gonorrhea, which attack the general health in addition to their deleterious effects on the reproductive system. They are very communicable diseases which should be treated by a medical doctor.

6. **Inherited Impotency:** There are some people born with inherent defects of the ovaries and testes. Since an infant receives its genes, physical characteristics, and innate energy from its parents, unhealthy parents can cycle their weaknesses down to the next generation. Unfortunately, inherited impotency is often permanent, but it is also very rare.

Ways to Strengthen Potency

There are as many ways to recharge the kidneys as there are to deplete them. Emotional work that encourages openness, trust, communication, and the willingness to let go of expectations and judgments can greatly improve interpersonal problems, including sexual ones. Ways to srengthen potency by improving physical health include a routine practice of Acu-Yoga, regular exercise, and a healthy balanced diet.

---

[39] Wilhelm Baynes, *The I Ching*, page 129.

Diet has an important role to play because the sexual hormones are affected by the foods we eat. Imbalances of these hormones can contribute to impotency and a lack of sexual appetite. For example, a common Oriental folk remedy calls for a medicinal use of beans:

> *"Beans are sometimes use as a medicine, internally as well as externally. Azuki beans are excellent for kidney disorders. Black beans are good for the sexual organs, for example in cases of irregular menstruation, barrenness, and lack of sexual appetite."*[40]

Eating a combination of three parts grain to one part beans not only complements all of the essential amino acids for a complete protein, but also helps to stabilize the sexual hormones in both men and women.* A balanced diet of whole, fresh foods is necessary for good health, and is one of the most valuable elements in generating sexual potency.

There are also Acupressure points related to the kidneys that aid potency. Acupressure works to build overall health, and therefore potency. The points around the sacrum, for example, are helpful for building sexual potency in both women and men. They have been found to correct menstrual disorders and irregularities in the prostate and bladder. The following exercise, "Warming the Vitals," presses these points which stimulate the secretion of sex-related hormones for developing potency.

The exercises listed under Pelvic Tension, Indigestion, Spinal Disorders, Back Problems (especially the one for the lower back), Frustration, and Fatigue are also beneficial for balancing the conditions that contribute to impotency. Daily practice of the exercises along with a natural foods diet and outdoor exercise can strengthen your condition.

Warming the Vitals

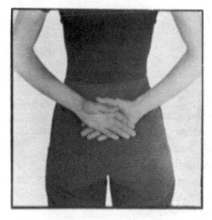

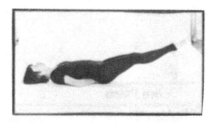

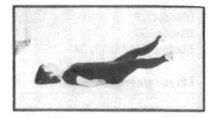

1. Lie on your back. Place your hands, one on top of the other, under the sacrum at the base of the spine.

---

[40] Noboru Muramoto, *Healing Ourselves*, page 72.
* See the section "Indigestion" for some tips on preparing beans.

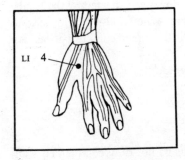

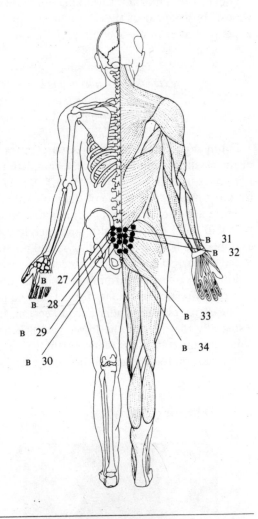

2. Inhale, raising the legs one foot off the ground. Exhale, keeping them up.

3. Inhale and spread your legs apart, still off the ground. Keep the legs straight.

4. Exhale and bring your legs together, still keeping them up one foot off the ground.

5. Continue for 20 seconds. Then relax on your back. Breathe deeply into your lower abdomen.

6. Repeat the exercise once more, relaxing for a few minutes afterwards.

Acu Points	Traditional Associations
Bladder 27	Disorders of the sacroiliac joint, colitis.
Bladder 28	Retention of urine, pain in lumbosacral area.
Bladder 29	Kidneys weak, back stiff, impotency.
Bladder 30	Lubago, sacral pain, sciatica.
Bladder 31, 32, 33, 34	Constipation, lumbago, impotency, sterility, vaginal discharge, genital diseases.
Large Intestine 4	Constipation, mental confusion, or obsession.

Benefits: constipation, lower back disorders, pain or pressure at the base of the spine, abdominal weakness, sciatica, bladder and sexual reproductive weaknesses.

Resistance to Illness

Our resistance to illness is in direct relationship with the balance, strength, and flexibility of our bodies. If we take care of ourselves by eating properly, getting enough rest and exercise, and by practicing techniques that release old tensions and blockages and balance our meridians—such as Acu-Yoga, meditation, Acupressure or Tai Chi Chuan—then our resistance to illness is strong. If, on the other hand, we abuse our bodies, push ourselves too hard, eat badly, don't exercise, and don't involve ourselves with practices that release tension and balance our energy, our resistance will be low, or weak, and we will be more prone to illness.

Fatigue is an important element in your resistance level. In this fast-paced society it is easy to overwork yourself, to take on too many commitments, to push yourself beyond your limits and into fatigue. This imbalance has a weakening effect on all parts of the body.

When we get enough rest, however, we give our bodies a chance to fully recover from our activities. Deep relaxation furthers the circulation of both blood and Ki in nourishing the whole body, especially the internal organs.

Dietary Considerations

Diet also plays an important role in resistance to illness. When we eat processed, preserved, or devitalized foods, we weaken our system and our resistance. However, foods that "yangize," or strengthen, the body build resistance, reinforcing the body's ability to protect itself. Examples are miso soup, parsley, beans, tofu, sea vegetables, sautéed vegetables, and lightly toasted sesame seeds.

Acupressure Points

There is a particular Acupressure point, Bladder 36, that governs resistance, especially resistance to colds and flus. It is located near the spine off the tips of the shoulder blades. The Chinese book, *The Yellow Emperor's Classic of Internal Medicine* says, "wind and cold enter the pores of the skin"[41] at this point. It, as well as other points in this area, helps to strengthen the body's resistance. The opposite is also true in that these points around the tips of the shoulder blades are the first to get blocked up just before an illness, especially a cold or flu, takes hold.

An ancient Indian method for maintaining resistance against illness is to swing a thick branch or club back and forth. The Yogis would do this when they felt any illness about to come on, since it was common knowledge that the tensions which accumulate between the shoulder blades contribute to illness. The swinging motion helped break down this tension. Swinging a baseball bat around moves and stretches the shoulder blades to release the tensions that collect there.

The following pose, "Yoga Mudra (Variation No. 3)," works on these same points, directly pressing them as the shoulder blades are brought together. Shoulder Stand (page

---

[41] Felix Mann, *Treatment of Disease by Acupuncture*, pages 32, 37.

224) and Plow Pose (page 136) are also excellent postures for releasing these tensions and developing resistance.

Yoga Mudra

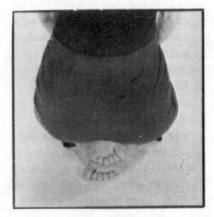

1. Sit on your heels, bringing the instep of one foot into the arch of the other.
2. Lower your head slowly forward to the ground.
3. With your arms behind your back, interlock your fingers (palms facing each other).
4. Inhale and raise your arms straight up, keeping your hands clasped. Breathe deeply in this position for 30 to 60 seconds.
5. Inhale and stretch the arms a little further; exhale and slowly lower them, release your hands, and let your arms relax on the floor, palms up. Relax in this position for a couple of minutes.

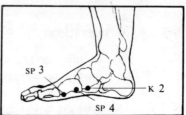

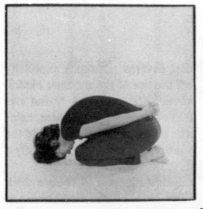

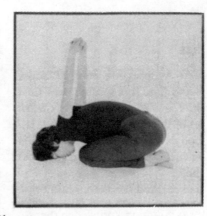

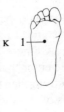

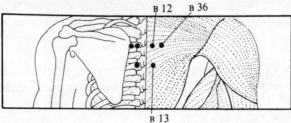

Acu Points	Traditional Associations
Bladder 12	Prevention and after-effects of chills, flu, fever.
Bladder 13	Cough, chest feels heavy, lung congested, pneumonia, agitation, boredom.
Bladder 36	Where "wind and cold enter the pores of the skin."
Spleen 3, 4	Fever, body heavy, cold feet, upset stomach.
Kidney 1, 2	Sore throat, head feels congested, cold or damp feet.

Benefits: resistance to illness, the lungs, skin, pressures, pain, or tightness in the upper back, poor circulation into the hands, shoulder tension.

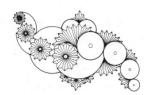

Shoulder Tension

Shoulder tension is a general indicator of a person's overall body tension, blockages, and stagnation. Many of the meridians that run through the arms, back, and neck cross in the shoulder region. When we are under stress or in danger, we automatically hunch our shoulders. This is a survival reflex which serves to protect the exposed neck and the head. Unfortunately, these days this instinctual mechanism contributes to chronic shoulder tension. This is why shoulder and neck tensions are the first symptoms that appear when the body is under stress.

Cultural Causes

Modern life styles contribute to shoulder tension. Sedentary living, such as watching TV for recreation and the use of cars for transportation, causes lethargy and restricts the mobility of the entire body, including the shoulders.

Many jobs today also create and reinforce shoulder tensions. Typing, working at a desk or over a machine or computer can cause shoulder tension. As your posture slumps, your breathing gets shallow, and tensions develop. Truck drivers who hunch their shoulders as they hold the wheel develop these tensions. People who do close work, such as electronics, graphic arts, needlework, and jewelry-making have a similar problem. Anyone in competitive, stressful situations, whether executive or student, usually suffers from shoulder tension.

Less industrialized cultures used their bodies more than we do simply for survival. The physical labor of working with the earth, hunting, and the play of active games and dancing kept their muscles in shape. Now that we are freed from the harshness of a survival existence, it is up to each one of us to provide the activity and relaxation that no longer is a part of our daily lives.

Emotional Causes

Shoulder tension can also be the result of emotional stresses and strains. These can easily build up, causing chronic problems. The feeling of "carrying the world on your shoulders" is literally true. The pressures of obligations, guilt, and burdensome responsibilities do rest heavily on the shoulder area. As a result, the trapezius muscles can become tight and rigid. This tension itself then contributes to uptightness and irritability, which are also related to shoulder tension.

When feelings are not expressed, they are stored in the body instead. Most of us retain a lot of old emotional stress in our bodies, which limits us both physically and emotionally. Toxins build up physically; fears, worries, anger, anxiety build up emotionally. We block our great natural capacity that comes from the mind and body working together. This is one way the innate homeostatic balancing mechanism is thrown off balance.

Most people unconsciously avoid parts of their bodies. People tend to block part of themselves off to escape painful past experiences that have internalized physically. By releasing shoulder tensions, emotions often surface that the person is not used to experiencing and handling. In the beginning it can seem like opening a Pandora's Box of problems, as buried emotions—fears, anger, hurts—begin to surface. However, the release of these buried emotions frees us incredibly from the old emotional baggage that we've been carrying around. Releasing shoulder tensions and their associated emotions can be an important part of a growth process for experiencing more aliveness, more wholeness, a fresh sense of things.

Physical Associations

The shoulder girdle is designed for motion, adjusting to movements of the arms and back. The structure of the shoulder girdle is like that of the yoke which Hollanders used to carry their water pails, parallel to the ground. If one shoulder is higher than another, there is an imbalance.

Three parts of the trapezius muscle govern the shoulder area. This very strong muscle reinforces the shoulder from the ligaments attached to the skull and the vertebrae of the neck and upper back. The shoulders structurally also gain support from the sternum. The muscles of the shoulder area extend out in all directions, like the spokes of a wheel, coordinating movement of the arms, neck, head, and upper body.[42]

Shoulder tensions, therefore, also affect all these parts of the body. They block off circulation to the extremities, directly for the arms, and indirectly (through the balance of the upper and lower spine) for the legs. Both blood and Ki flow are restricted, often causing cold hands and feet. By releasing shoulder tension, a wave of warmth can be released into the extremities.

---

[42] Mabel E. Todd, *The Thinking Body*, pages 143–157.

Fatigue is another problem associated with shoulder tension, since it blocks the flow of blood and Ki, causing a lack of energy or sluggishness. You may wish to practice the exercise listed for the section on "Fatigue" as well as the ones here, since it also works to release shoulder tension. Through Acu-Yoga exercises, shoulder tensions can be released. A new sense of vitality and rejuvenation can emerge. Balancing this area has strong effects on the entire body, and is a key part of an overall body release.

Quick Hints for Shoulder Tension

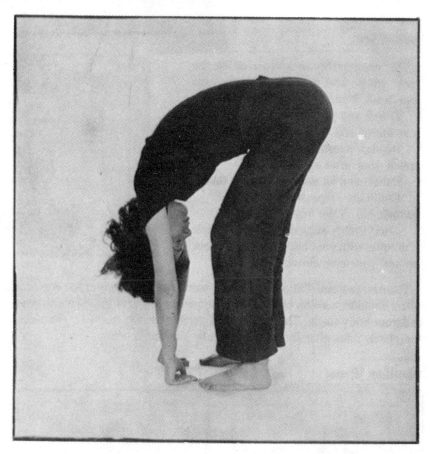

"Ragdoll"

1. Stand with your feet comfortably apart.

2. Exhale and slowly drop your head forward, and then gradually let your body drop forward, following the head. Allow your head to hang with your neck relaxed. Let your arms droop and dangle.

3. Begin long deep breathing in this position.

4. Continue for one minute. Really let go!

5. Slowly come up to a standing position. Close your eyes for a minute and let yourself relax to discover the benefits.

Reflexology

Sit comfortably and massage the feet, especially the outside areas. Press in between the bones on the tops of the feet. Also press the reflex point for the shoulders, located on the bottom of the foot, a finger's width below the little toe.

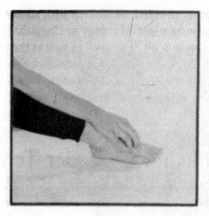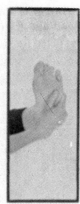

Isometrics

1. Sit comfortably in a chair or on the floor. Inhale and bring your arms over your head. Interlock your fingers.
2. Exhale and pull your arms apart with your fingers still interlocked.
3. Inhale, releasing the lock as you stretch your arms upwards.
4. Exhale and let your arms relax down.
5. Continue, repeating steps No. 2 through No. 4 for one minute.
6. Comfortably sit straight for a couple of minutes with your hands resting in your lap and your eyes closed.

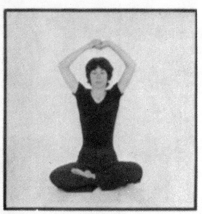

The next exercise, "Shoulder Press," works on Gall Bladder 21, one of the major points where shoulder tension collects. It is so powerful that it might make your head feel light and your body tingle. That is a good sign that tension has been released. Make sure you completely relax after the exercise to fully gain the benefits.

Shoulder Press

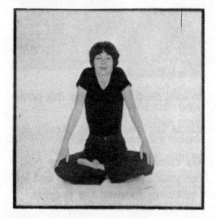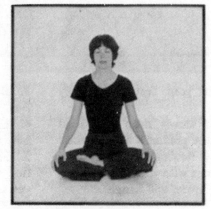

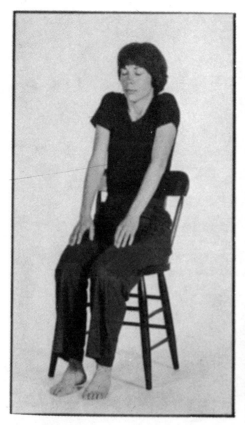 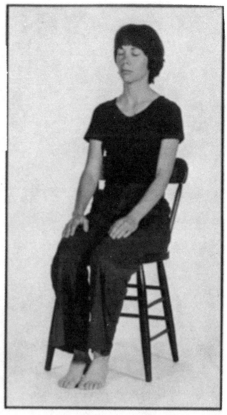

1. Sit comfortably with your hands on your knees.

2. Inhale, raising the shoulders firmly pressing them up toward the ears.

3. Exhale and let the shoulders drop down.

4. Continue for one minute, inhaling up and exhaling down, slowly building speed and keeping the rhythm steady.

5. Inhale, press the shoulders up and hold the breath for 10 seconds.

6. Relax on your back for a few minutes to discover the benefits.

The Acupressure points and associations for this exercise are the same as those for "Bridge Pose." Please see the next page for the chart and illustration.

Benefits: tense, arching shoulders, rheumatism, uptightness, frustration, depression, lack of motivation, repressed anger, stiff neck.

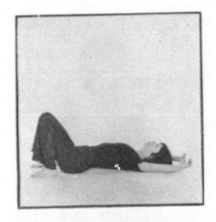

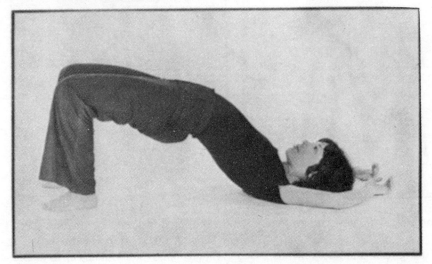

Bridge Pose

1. Lie on your back.
2. Bend your knees so that the soles of your feet are flat on the floor.
3. Put your arms above your head on the floor and relax them.
4. Inhale, arching the pelvis up. Hold for several seconds.
5. Exhale as you slowly come down. Continue to inhale up and exhale down for one minute.
6. Relax on your back with your eyes closed for a few minutes.

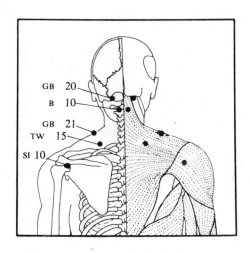

Acu Points	Traditional Associations
Triple Warmer 15	Shoulder and neck pain, arm and elbow painful and cannot be raised, stiff neck.
Gall Bladder 20	Alternately hot and cold, eyes foggy, nervousness, painful shoulder, rheumatism, stiff neck, upper parts of the body feel heavy or hot.
Gall Bladder 21	The major point where shoulder tension collects. Traditionally used to release stiff neck, regulate hyperthyroidism, and relieve rheumatism.
Bladder 10	Head heavy, spasm of the neck muscles, limbs and body not coordinated, throat sore or swollen.
Small Intestine 10	Muscular pain, numbness, swelling or arthritis in the shoulder—scapula region.

Benefits: fatigue, cold hands or feet, nervous exhaustion, irritability, shoulder pain or ache, excessive anger, hypertension, resistance to colds and flu.

The last exercise, "Shoulder Stand," is an inverted posture which reverses the pull of gravity on the body. The blood flows more easily to the heart in this position. The head and neck are flushed with a fresh flow of blood, nourishing the thyroid, tonsils, thalamus, and neck muscles. The Yogis teach that 15 minutes in shoulder stand is equal to two full hours of sleep. Beginners should start with one minute, building the time gradually.

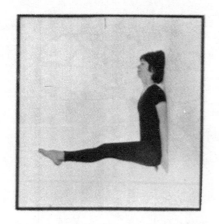

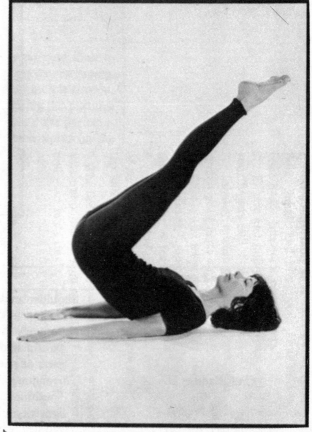

Shoulder Stand

1. Lie on your back, hands at your sides.
2. On an exhalation, lift the legs up, and when they are straight up, push off with your arms to lift the trunk of your body up. Use your hands to support your back.
3. Breathe long and deep in this position for one minute. Allow your body to relax in this posture so that your weight will naturally press your shoulders into the ground.
4. Put your arms back on the floor and slowly lower yourself down.
5. Relax on your back with your eyes closed for a few minutes.

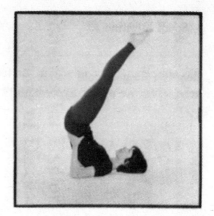

The Acupressure points and traditional associations for this pose are the same as those listed in the previous exercise.

Benefits: the brain, foggy thinking, hypo-thyroid, nervous disorders, arm problems, learning disabilities, sore throat, resistance to colds and flus.

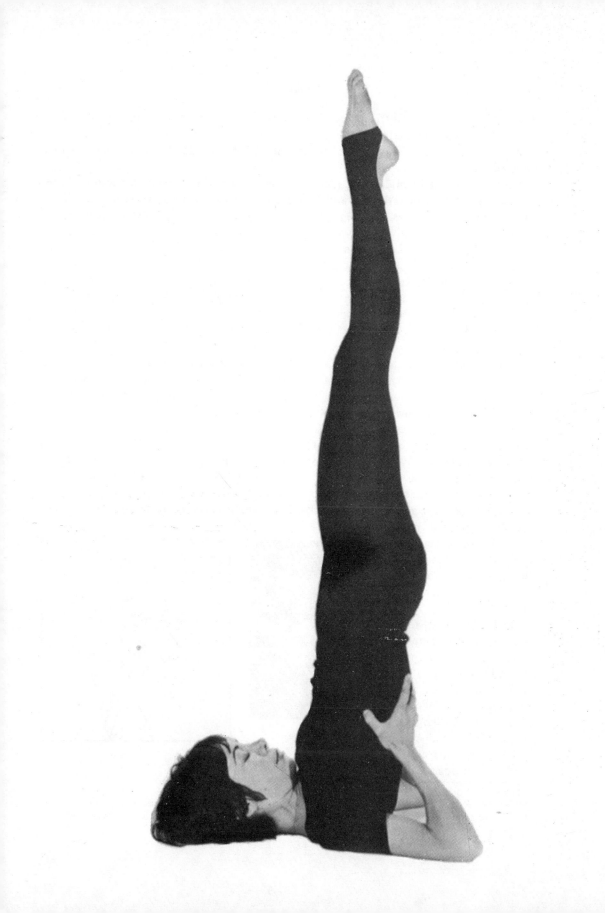

Sinuses

The sinuses are cavities which surround the nose and eyes. When fluids in the back of the nose are blocked and unable to drain, pressure builds up in the sinus areas. If this condition is not relieved eventually the swollen membranes inside the sinuses can become infected.

There is little use in eradicating such symptoms of sinusitis as nasal congestion, headache, and pressure around the eyes and the bridge of the nose without exploring the original causes for these symptoms. Although there are Acupressure techniques which benefit sinus conditions, it is imperative that you go beyond a symptomatic release to discover and eliminate the causes of the problem, so that you can prevent their reoccurrence.*

In many cases, sinus problems are caused by emotional holding, such as grief or fear. This holding can also cause muscular tension in the chest, which blocks the descending flows. (In this case, hold the Acupressure points along the pectoralis muscles on the chest with firm, prolonged pressure.) Once a person uses Acupressure to release this tension, repressed emotions can surface and be dealt with directly, enabling the nasal passages of the sinuses to clear.

Constipation, poor dietary habits, and lack of exercise are also contributing factors.** An experiment that you can try is to abstain from all dairy products for a few weeks, and see if your sinus condition improves. You can also try massaging the reflexology points for sinuses, which are on the sides and bottoms of the toes.

Structurally the sinuses resemble pockets or valleys. The Acupressure point that is traditionally recommended for treatment of the sinuses is Large Intestine 4,*** the "joining of the valleys." As the governor of the descending meridians, Large Intestine 4 can help to open up and drain the sinuses. Bladder 2 at the bridge of the nose is also a helpful Acupressure point for frontal headaches and sinus conditions. On the skull, Governing Vessel 20 and Bladder 7 are additional points that have also been traditionally used to help open

up the congested nasal passages. Large Intestine 20 and Stomach 3 on the face are the foremost points for the maxillary sinuses located in the cheek areas.

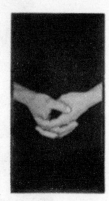

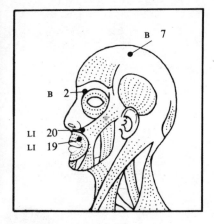

Remember that this represents a more symptomatic approach and that you must look beyond the symptom of sinuses to discover the cause of your discomfort. The following Acu-Yoga pose, "Drilling Bamboo," helps work on the Acupressure points mentioned above, to relieve sinus problems.

---

* See the "Meditation for Exploring the Cause of Disease."
** See the sections on "Constipation" and "Indigestion" for more information.
*** Please refer to the "Squat Pose" on page 144 which presses an important point for relieving headaches.

Drilling Bamboo

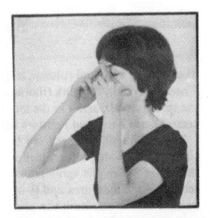

1. Lie on your back. Bend your knees, so that your feet are flat on the floor near the buttocks, about 1-1/2 feet apart.

2. Place your index fingers into the points underneath the ridge at the inside top of the eye. Your third finger will rest lightly on the Third Eye, between the eyebrows. Use your thumbs to hold your jaw muscles and then move them to the hollow indentation of your temples.

3. Inhale, lifting your hips up off the ground. Breathe long and deep for one minute.

4. Then exhale and slowly come down.

5. Make fists and pound or massage the chest muscles.

6. Lie flat on the floor with your hands by your sides, your lips together and your eyes closed. Completely relax your entire body.

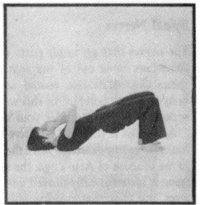

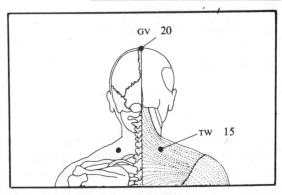

Acu Points	Traditional Associations
Bladder 2 and 7	Hay fevers, sinusitis, allergies, sneezing, headaches.
Triple Warmer 15 and Governing Vessel 20	Shoulder pain or tension, chest heavy, troubled, melancholia.
Large Intestine 19 and 20	Sinusitis, facial paralysis, nose blocked.

Benefits: shoulder, neck and eye tensions, flus, hay fever, allergies, sinusitis, facial paralysis, headaches.

227

Spinal Disorders

The spine, or vertebral column, is the keystone of the body. It is composed of 33 vertebrae: 7 neck (cervical), 12 trunk (thoracic), 5 lower back (lumbar), 5 fused bones at the base of the spine (sacral), and 4 in the tail bone (coccyx). It supports the entire body, protects the central nerve cord, and registers the youth and health of a person.

The individual vertebrae can become misaligned either from muscular tension, emotional stress, poor posture, lack of movement, falls or accidents, or the misalignment of the pelvis. When the spine is out of alignment a negative cycle begins, creating muscle tension in the local area and in other parts of the back, which must work harder to compensate for the strain on the primary area.

Spinal Nerves

The nerves that go to all parts of the body and control all our organs, functions, and sensations come out of the spinal nerve cord. It is of utmost importance to keep our spines aligned, flexible, strong, and balanced since this master nerve is housed inside the bony vertebral column. In this way the condition of the spine affects the condition of the entire body. The healthier your spine is, the healthier your whole body is.

Acu-Yoga is the most effective form of self-treatment for spinal disorders. These time-tested, scientific exercises work the spine in all directions to promote flexibility and strength. In the practice of Acu-Yoga, the spine often adjusts itself naturally as each vertebra of the spine is systematically moved and stretched. This prevents uneven pressure on the spinal discs, the pads that cushion and separate the individual vertebrae. Immobility and inflexibility of the spine, along with poor posture, result in spinal misalignments, degeneration of the discs, and pinched nerves.

Misalignment

The physicians of ancient Greece and Rome, as well as those of the East, recognized the importance of the spine in maintaining health. Many of these physicians, after studying the postures, positions, and irregularities of the spine worked with exercises and manipulations to correct structural problems which often affect the rest of the body.

Nowadays, we have chiropractors who adjust the spine to correct spinal and other problems. Chiropractic work and Acu-Yoga go hand in hand. If a person has a chiropractic adjustment to align his or her spine, the benefits will last longer if that person follows up by practicing Acu-Yoga to keep the spine flexible and in alignment. Conversely, if a person who practices Acu-Yoga receives a chiropractic adjustment, the adjustment will be easier in that (1) the muscles will have better tone, and therefore will not hold the spine out of position so strongly, and not resist the manipulation, and (2) there should be fewer misalignments, and the ones present should be of a smaller magnitude, compared to someone who does not do Acu-Yoga.

The Governing Vessel: The Master of the Spine

One of the most important Acupressure meridians, the Governing Vessel (GV), runs directly over the spine. This meridian and the spine strongly influences each other's overall strength and balance. Keeping the spine flexible and strong has a direct and positive effect on the GV, and keeping the flow of energy in the GV strong has a beneficial effect on the spinal column and central nerve cord. Similarly, a problem in one can cause a problem in the other, as is shown in the following quote:

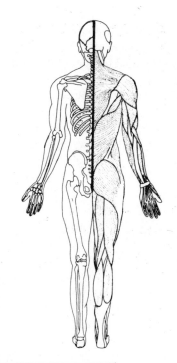

"When the [Governing Vessel] meridian is overactive, the spine becomes stiff, as the meridian Qi [energy] is blocked."[43]

Spinal pain

Because the nerves from the spine go to all parts of the body, some people suffer from referred pains which run from the back along the sides or other parts of the body. Movement in a certain direction or deep breathing (which moves the ribs that are connected to the spine) may stimulate these pains in various areas. Often a spinal problem in the back will cause a referred pain in the front of the body, opposite the original problem.

The last two ribs can get pushed out of place especially easily. These 11th and 12th ribs— the "floating ribs"—are not attached to the sternum, and a strong impact or twist can put them out of place, causing a shock to the nerves and the discs associated with these ribs.

By practicing Acu-Yoga, you can improve the condition of your spine, and of your muscles and organs as well. Daily practice promotes longevity and enhances the beauty of the face and body. The following two exercises work on the Governing Vessel, and the "Spinal Flex" especially stimulates the spinal nerve cord which branches out down from the brain. This nerve cord is protected in the bony vertebrae by three layers of membranes and the cerebrospinal fluid that flows between them, which also flows through the brain itself. The "Spinal Flex" exercise flexes and extends the spine back and forth, gently stretching the spinal muscles that hold the vertebrae in place. This enables the cerebrospinal fluid to circulate freely, and improves the condition of the spine and of the back

---

[43] Felix Mann, *The Meridians of Acupuncture*, page 112.

muscles. Traditionally, Yogis were able to prevent many types of spinal curvatures (scoliosis) through these exercises.

The second exercise, "Cobra Pose," stretches the spine to increase its flexibility, release tension, and prevent scoliosis. It stimulates the nerves of the back to blance all the internal organs. "Cobra Pose" is also good for nervousness, headaches, hypertension, impatience, and sexual imbalances.

> *"An abundant flow of blood reaches the backbone and sympathetic nerves in Cobra Pose . . . . The kidneys, too, are regenerated and given an abundant supply of blood. In India this Asana is used chiefly to prevent calculus formations in the kidneys (kidney stones). During the exercise, the blood is squeezed out of the kidneys, but as soon as the body returns to its original position, a vigorous flow of blood invades them and washes away any deposits. The thyroid gland is stimulated and any functional disturbances are corrected . . . . This exercise is also useful in developing self-confidence and overcoming inferiority complexes."*[44]

Please read the previous sections on "The Flexibility of the Spine," page 34, and on "Back Problems." They include important information and exercises that anyone with a spinal disorder should know about and utilize for better understanding of the back and spine.

Spinal Flex

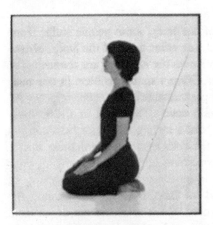 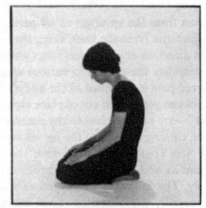

1. Sit on the heels, placing the top of the right foot over the arch of the left foot.
2. Place the palms on the thighs, with the spine straight.

3. Inhale and flex your spine forward. Arch the spine gently but firmly in this motion.
4. Exhale and let the spine slump back.

---

[44] Selvarajan Yesudian, *Yoga and Health*, pages 137–138.

This stretches the spine in the opposite direction. Let your head simply rest on your neck, moving slightly with each flex of the back.

5. Continue for one minute. Begin slowly and gradually, feeling the motion and stretch in your back. Gradually increase speed as your back loosens up. Breathe with each movement, inhaling as the chest pushes open and forward, and exhaling back and down.

6. Completely relax on your back for a couple of minutes.

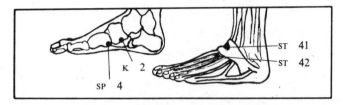

Acu Points	Traditional Associations
Spleen 4	A reflex point for the mid-upper back, digestive problems, abdominal pain.
Kidney 2	A reflex point for the middle of the back, cold feet, chest or abdominal pain, swelling.
Stomach 41, 42	Always cold, walks around aimlessly, vertigo, madness, fits.
Governing Vessel 1–16	Back stiff and painful, loins and spine rigid, nervousness.

Cobra Pose

1. Lie on your stomach with your feet together and your chin on the floor. Place your palms on the ground underneath your shoulders.

2. Inhale slowly, lifting your head up and stretching the cervical vertebrae of the neck. Continue inhaling, and raise the chest, using both the arms and the back muscles.

3. Finish the inhalation and arch all the way up. Your hips will be on the ground, your arms may be either bent or straight,

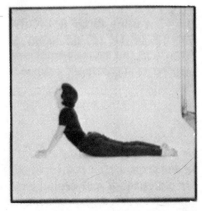

depending upon the flexibility of your spine.

4. Exhale in this position, and begin long deep breathing for about 30 seconds, gently pressing the navel to the floor.

5. Using your arms for support, lower yourself part-way down so that the segment of the spine that needs the most attention recieves some pressure. Hold the body at this angle, breathing deeply into the blockage in the spine for another 30 seconds.

6. Slowly come down all the way, letting your head rest on its side, and your arms by your sides. Close your eyes and completely relax for several minutes.

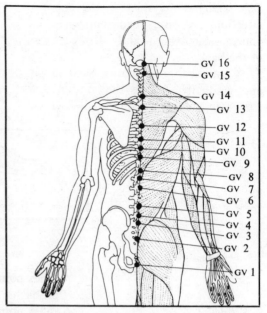

This pose should be followed by an exercise that stretches the spine in the opposite direction, such as the "Life Nerve Stretch," or "Plow Pose." People with spinal problems should always use common sense about what and how much exercise is appropriate for them. Practice Cobra and Plow Pose with care and always let yourself completely relax after each exercise to obtain the benefits.

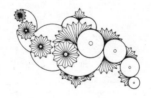

Acu Points	Traditional Associations	Area of the spine that Benefits	Approximate No. of inches from the Ground and Position
Governing Vessel 15, 16	Neck stiff, rigid, headache, colds, speech problems, fear, suicidal.	Cervical (neck)	3–5 inches head back
Governing Vessel 11, 12, 13, 14	Nervousness, spine rigid and painful, eyes heavy, neck, shoulders and back painful.	Upper Thoracic (upper back)	6–9 inches arching chest out
Governing Vessel 6, 7, 8, 9, 10	Back pain, lower back especially stiff, limbs weak, hypertension, cardiac pains.	Lower Thoracic (middle back)	10–12 inches 1/2 way up
Governing Vessel 4, 5	Lumbar pain, impotence, vaginal discharge, loins and back stiff and painful.	Lumbars (lower back)	12–15 inches almost completely up
Governing Vessel 1, 2, 3	Lower back painful, extreme nervousness, irregular periods, lumbago, colitis, abdominal distension.	Sacrum (small of the back)	15–18 inches all the way up & buttocks contracted

Benefits: bladder, kidneys, general back problems, nervous disorders and weakness, headaches.

Glossary

Acupressure: A method of bodywork that uses the Chinese system of acupuncture points and meridians combined with Japanese finger pressure techniques to release muscular tensions.

Acupuncture: A traditional method of Chinese medicine in which fine needles are inserted into the body in key points to release internal blockages and balance energy.

Acu-Yoga: An integration of Acupressure and Yoga used for self-treatment.

Affirmations: Personal statements said aloud or thought to oneself that positively validates different aspects of one's existence. They are used to creatively enable one to visualize and increase the benefits of Acu-Yoga techniques.

Aikido: A Japanese art of self-defense using the momentum of your opponent's energy while remaining centered.

Apana: A form of prana or vital force used for elimination.

Asanas: Traditional yoga postures.

Ayurveda: An ancient healing system developed in India based on the three humors: fire, mucus, and wind.

Blockage: An accumulation or congestion of energy in or surrounding an Acupressure point. Blockages in a meridian may ache, be painful, or feel numb before manifesting as a physical symptom.

Breathing awareness: The ability to deepen and direct the breath into different parts of the body through concentration and relaxation.

Centering: The process of gaining awareness of the mind and body. This enables a person to be more conscious in the present moment.

Chakra: A vital center for giving and receiving life energy. Chakras are anatomically identified with the nerve plexuses of the body.

Chi: A Chinese word for vital energy. It has been translated as "material energy" or "vital matter" which circulates through the meridians.

Ching Chi: The reserved energy stored in the kidneys.

Chronic muscular tension: A long term condition in which the muscle fibers are held indefinitely in a shortened, contracted state.

Deep Relaxation: The letting go of all parts of the body and mind to allow a natural flow of energy to circulate in its natural course. To completely relax after strenuous exercise is the best way to recharge the nervous system.

Disease: An imbalance in the system as a whole.

Dō-In: Methods of self-acupressure.

Energy: The basis of all forms of life and matter in the universe. It is a dynamic force that circulates through the body in specific pathways called meridians.

Energy blockage: An obstruction to the free flow of vital matter which manifests physically as tension, pain, or stiffness. Thoughts and emotions can also cause energy blockages.

The Five Elements: Wood, fire, earth, water, and metal.

Grounded: The experience of being connected with the Earth.

Guru: A teacher for spiritual guidance.

Hatha Yoga: Unification of the body through postures and deep relaxation. Hatha literally means "sun-moon."

Holistic: An approach to life based on a perspective that all forms of existence are unified, that the whole equals more than the sum of its parts and that every aspect, whether internal or external, affects the whole.

Homeostatic: A mechanism of equilibrium or balance.

Hypertension: Abnormally high arterial blood pressure.

Hyperventilation: Heavy breathing through the mouth, which results in an excessive intake of oxygen and elimation of carbon dioxide from the blood, causing nausea or extreme dizziness.

Ida: One of the sympathetic channels which lies parallel and outside of the spinal cord. The ida governs yin energy.

Impotence: The inability to have satisfying sexual relationships. Unusual vaginal discharge or premature ejaculation can be preliminary signs of developing impotence.

The Infinite: Unlimited scope or potential.

Intuition: The inner guidance of meaningful thought and impressions.

Jin Shin: A highly developed Acupressure massage technique which uses gentle-to-deep finger pressure applied to specific points on the human anatomy. This system releases tension and rebalances all areas of the body.

Karma: The universal law of cause and affect.

Karma Yoga: Purifying one's actions through service.

Ki: The Japanese word for the vital life energy which concentrates in all living things. It circulates through the human body in pathways called meridians.

Kundalini: The energy that resides in the base of the spine which can be activated upward for spiritual reawakening.

Life Force: The vital energy contained in all things. The three main types are:
(1) the energy that circulates through the body via the meridians.
(2) the power generated from the human qualities of love, devotion, determination, willpower and positive thinking or projection; and
(3) the forces of nature which include the wind, rain, sun, heat, magnetism, gravity, and electricity.

Lumbar: The last five vertebrae before the sacrum on the lower back.

Mantra: Sounds which are used repeatedly during meditation to affect higher states of consciousness.

Medial: At the center of the body.

Meditation: Focussing one's attention for developing the spiritual capabilities of the mind.

Meridians: The pathways along which Ki energy flows through the body, connecting the various Acupressure/Acupuncture points and the internal organs.

Yin Meridians		Yang Meridians	
Lung	Lu	Large Intestine	LI
Spleen	Sp	Stomach	St
Heart	H	Small Intestine	SI
Kidney	K	Bladder	B
Pericardium	P	Triple Warmer	TW
Liver	Lv	Gall Bladder	GB
Conception Vessel	CV	Governing Vessel	GV

Movement Therapy: Utilizing dance and creative movements as a form of self healing.

Mudras: Acu-Yoga postures which produce electrical currents through the meridians.

Nervous System: The network of nerves which regulates muscular functioning. It influences the coordination of every cell, organ, and system in the body with one's environment.

Nei Ching, The Yellow Emperor's Classic of Internal Medicine: An important traditional Chinese medical book written in 2697 B.C. by Huang Ti, the Yellow Emperor.

Prana: The essential life force which circulates in the air, food, plants, and in the human body. It is the life behind the atom, found in all forms of matter, and is concentrated in living things.

Pranayama: The science of controlling the breath. It is used in Acu-Yoga to increase the effectiveness of exercises.

Pressure points: Places on the human anatomy with high levels of electrical conductivity. They tend to be located in neuro-muscular junctions, in the joints, or where bone lies close to the skin along a meridian.

Referred Pain: Pain generated in one area of the body but felt in another.

Regulatory Channels: The eight pathways that link all of the organ meridians together. Acu-Yoga stimulates these channels, and the relaxation which follows the exercises serves to balance them.

Shiatsu: A Japanese form of Acupressure which uses various finger pressure massage techniques on points along the meridians.

Spinal Column: The backbone, composed of a series of bones called vertebrae, which are stacked on top of one another.

Stress: Tensions which tend to disturb the body's natural balance when internalized.

Tai Chi Chuan: A traditional Chinese system of movement which enables the body to balance and maintain health.

Tao: Ancient Chinese principle based on the oneness of the Universe. Taoism emphasizes the unity of humanity and nature, the relativity of all things.

Tofu: A traditional Oriental food made from soybeans.

Tonic: A technique or substance that invigorates the whole system.

Tsubo: The Japanese word for Acupressure point.

Visualization: A creative process of forming images and thoughts which positively directs one's life.

Wei Chi: Protective body energy.

Yin and Yang: The two polar forces which interact on all levels of existence, creating constant change.

> **Yang**—is the active or contractive force
> **Yin**—is the passive or expansive force

Yoga: "Union." Yoga utilizes various ancient techniques to bring about a natural balance of body and mind.

Yoga Postures: Body positions which stretch and strengthen the spine, limbs, joints, and muscles as well as tones the glands and nerves.

Yogic Sleep: A deep healing state achieved through Yoga that naturally rebalances the meridians. In this state, a person remains conscious of the present and at the same time experiences realms out of the body. The most profound healing can naturally take place at this time.

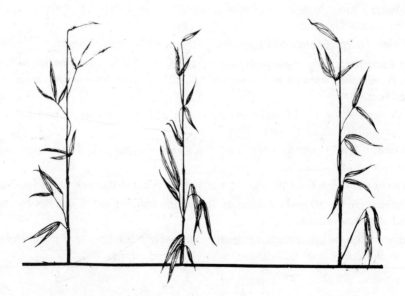

Bibliography

Academy of Traditional Chinese Medicine. *An Outline of Chinese Acupuncture*. Peking: Foreign Languages Press, 1975.

Adidevananda, Swami. *Yoga as a Therapeutic Fact*. Mysore, India: University of Mysore, 1966.

Baker, Douglas, M.D. *Esoteric Anatomy*. Little Elephant, Kentish Lane, Herts, England. Published by the author, 1976.

Ballentine, Rudolph M. (Editor). *Science of Breath*. Glenview, Illinois. The Himalayan International Institute of Yoga Science and Philosophy of U.S.A., 1977.

A Barefoot Doctor's Manual. Prepared by the Revolutionary Health Committee of Hunan Province. Seattle, Washington: Cloudburst Press, 1977.

Bean, Roy E., M.D. *Helping Your Health with Pointed Pressure Therapy*. West Nyack, New York: Parker Publishing Company, 1975.

Beau, Georges. *Chinese Medicine*. New York, New York: Avon Books, 1972.

Bendix, G. *Press Point Therapy*. New York, New York: Avon Books, 1976.

Brena, Steven F., M.D. *Yoga and Medicine*. New York, New York: Penguin Books, 1973.

Brodsky, Greg. *From Eden to Aquarius*. New York, New York: Bantam Books, 1974.

Chang, Stephan. *Complete Book of Acupuncture*. Millbrae, California: Celestial Arts, 1976.

Chao, Pi Chen. *Taoist Yoga*. Translated by Ku'an Yu Lu. New York, New Ycrk: Weiser, 1970.

Cannon, Walter B., M.D. *The Wisdom of the Body*. New York, New York: W. W. Norton and Company, 1963.

Carr, Rachel. *The Yoga Way To Release Tension*. New York, New York: Harper & Row, Publishers, 1975.

Carter, Mildred. *Helping Yourself with Foot Reflexology*. West Nyack, New York: Parker Publishing Company, 1969.

Chen, Ronald. *The History and Methods of Physical Diagnosis in Classical Chinese Medicine*. New York, New York: Vantage Press, 1969.

Desai, Yogi Shanti. *The Complete Practice Manual of Yoga*. Ocean City, New Jersey: Shanti Yogi Institute, 1976.

Feldenkrais, Moshe. *Awareness through Movement: Exercises for Personal Growth*. New York, New York: Harper & Row, 1972.

Garde, Raghanath K. M.D. *Principles and Practice of Yoga Therapy*. Lakemont, Georgia: Tarnhelm, 1970.

Geba, Bruno. *Breathe Away Your Tension: An Introduction to Gestalt Body Awareness Therapy*. New York, New York: Random House, 1974.

Heroldova, Dana. *Acupuncture and Moxibustion* (2 Volumes). Prague Academia, 1968.

Inayat Khan, Hazrat. *Book of Health*. London, England: Sufi Publishing Company, 1974.

Inayat Khan, Hazrat. *Practice of Sufi Healing*. New York, New York: Rainbow Bridge, 1977.

Iyengar, B.K.S. *Light on Yoga*. New York, New York: Schocker Books, 1966.

Jackson, Mildred, N.D., and Teague, Terri. *The Handbook of Alternatives to Chemical Medicine*. Berkeley, California: Bookpeople, 1975.

Kingsland, Kevin. *Complete Hatha Yoga*. New York, New York: Arco, 1976.

Kirschner, M. J. *Yoga for Health and Vitality*. Reading, Massachusetts: Allen & Unwin, 1977.

Kloss, Jethro. *Back to Eden*. New York, New York: Lancer Books, 1971.

Kundalini Research Institute. *Kundalini Yoga: Exercise and Meditation Manual*. Claremont, California: K.R.I. Publications, 1976.

Kushi, Michio. *The Teachings of Michio Kushi*. Boston, Massachusetts: East-West Foundation, 1972.

Langre, Jacques de. *Second Book of Do-In*. Magalia, California: Happiness Press, 1974.

Lappe, Frances Moore. *Diet for a Small Planet*. New York, New York: Ballantine, 1975.

Lawson-Wood, Denis and Joyce Lawson. *The Five Elements of Acupuncture and Chinese Massage*. Rustington, England: Health Science Press, 1965.

Leadbeater, C. W. *The Chakras*. Adyar, Madras 20, India: Theosophical Publishing House, 1969.

Lu, K'uan-Yu. *Secrets of Chinese Medicine*. New York, New York: Weiser, 1964.

Luce, Gay Gaer. *Biological Rhythms in Human & Animal Physiology*. New York, New York: Dover Publications, Inc., 1971.

Mann, Felix. *The Treatment of Disease by Acupuncture*. London, England: Heinemann Medical Books, Ltd., 1967.

Mann, Felix. *The Meridians of Acupuncture*. London, England: Heinemann Medical Books, Ltd., 1964.

Mann, Felix. *Acupuncture, The Ancient Chinese Art of Healing*. New York, New York: Random House, 1962.

Mann, Felix. *Atlas of Acupuncture*. Philadelphia, Pennsylvania: International Ideas, 1970.

Masunaga, Shizuto. *Zen Shiatsu*. Tokyo, Japan: Japan Publications, 1977.

Mishra, Rammurti. *Fundamentals of Yoga*. New York, New York: Lancer Books, 1959.

Muramoto, Noboru. *Healing Ourselves*. New York, New York: Avon Books, 1973.

Nutrition Search, Inc., *Nutrition Almanac*. New York, New York: McGraw-Hill Company, 1975.

Ohsawa, George. *Acupuncture and the Philosophy of the Far East*. Boston, Massachussetts: The Order of the Universe Publications, (Box 203, Prudential Center Station)

Oki, Masahiro. *Healing Yourself Through Okido Yoga*. Tokyo, Japan: Japan Publications, 1977.

Oki, Masahiro. *Practical Yoga*. Tokyo, Japan: Japan Publications, 1970.

Palos, Stephan. *The Chinese Art of Healing*. New York, New York: Bantam Books, 1972.

Rama, Swami. *Lectures on Yoga*. Chicago, Illinois: Himalayan International Institute of Yoga Science and Philosophy, 1976.

Ramacharaka, Yogi. *Science of Breath*. The Yogi Publication Society, 1905.

Rawls, Eugene and Diskin, Eve. *Yoga for Beauty and Health*. New York, New York:

Parker Publishing Company, 1967.

Samuels, Mike, M.D. and Bennett, Hal. *The Well Body Book*. New York, New York: Random House, 1975.

Saraswati, Srimat Swami Shivananda. *Yogic Therapy, The Yogic Way to Cure Diseases*. New York Agent, Samuel Weiser, 1964.

Satchidananda, Yogiraj Sri Swami. *Integral Yoga Hatha*. New York, New York: Holt, Rainehart and Winston, 1970.

Serizawa, Katsusuke, M.D. *Massage: The Oriental Method, Tsubo: Vital Points for Oriental Therapy*. Tokyo, Japan: Japan Publications, 1976.

Stevens, John O. *Awareness: Exploring, Experimenting, Experiencing*. Lafayette, California: Real People Press, 1971.

Thomson, Judi. *Healthy Pregnancy the Yoga Way*. Garden City, New York: Dolphin Books, Doubleday & Company 1977.

Thie, John F. *Touch for Health*. Marina Del Ray, California: De Vorss & Company, 1973.

Todd, Mabel Elsworth. *The Thinking Body*. New York, New York: Dance Horizons Republications, 1959.

Veith, Ilza (translated). Huang Ti Nei Ching Su Wen. Berkeley, California: University of California Press, 1949.

Vishnudevananda, Swami. *The Complete Illustrated Book of Yoga*. New York, New York: Bell Publishing Company, Inc., 1960.

Vithaldes, Yogi. *Yoga System of Health*. Birmingham, Alabama: Cornerstone, 1961.

Wallnofer and von Rottauscher. *Chinese Folk Medicine*. New York, New York: Crown Publishers, 1971.

White, Karen Cross. *Complete Sprouting Cookbook*. San Francisco, California: Troubador Press, 1975.

Wilhelm, Richard (translated), rendered into English by Cary Baynes, Princeton, New Hersey: Princeton University Press, 1968.

Yesudian, Selvarajan, and Elisabeth Haich. *Yoga and Health*. New York, New York: Harper & Row, 1965.

Yogananda, Paramahansa. *Scientific Healing Affirmations*. Los Angeles, California. Self-Realization Fellowship Publishers, 1974.

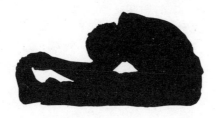

Index

holistic health, 15, 23, 124, 178
homeostatic, 17, 45, 79, 81
Huang-ti, 19
hundred meeting place—See thousand
petalled lotus
hypertension, 84, 126, 156, 167, 170, 178–
181, 204, 223, 233, See also blood pressure
hypothalamus, 81

I

I Ching, 80
imagination, 24, 37, 74, 164—See visualization
impotency, 65, 176, 207, 233
India, 23–25, 33
indigestion, 67, 130, 143, 144, 151,
164, 172, 176, 181–189, 205, 209, 213
inner peace, 17, 25, 29, 32, 38, 40
inner voice, 16, 24, 30, 31, 34
insomnia, 145, 190, 192, 196, 200, 205
instinct, 18
intellect, 17, 21, 23, 24, 74
internal nourishment, 41–43
internal organs, 16, 17, 19, 33, 36, 37, 61,
67, 71, 79, 95, 129, 136, 215
intestines, 126—See large intestines & small
intestines
intuition, 20, 23, 24, 30, 31
isometrics, 220

J, K

Jalandhara Bandha, 39
Jen Mo, 82
Jin Shin, 22, 173–175
jogging, 34
"joyful sleep" point, 191
karma, 26
Karma yoga, 21, 22
Ki energy, 15, 26, 37, 45, 80, 160, 161,
See also Chi energy
kidneys, 36, 61, 65, 67, 84, 88, 99, 111, 128,
130, 133, 148, 156, 176, 186, 192, 196,
204, 206, 210, 217, 231, 233
knee problems, 131, 137, 145
Kundalini yoga, 21, 39, 40

L

large intestine, 91, 99, 102, 103, 141, 145,
167, 172, 188, 190, 226, 227
Laya yoga, 21
leg problems, 131, 196
letting go, 38, 51
life nerve 35
life nerve stretch, 55, 129, 131

lifestyle, 16, 18, 20, 35, 202
lila, 25
liver, 40, 42, 56, 61, 67, 99, 117, 148, 149,
151, 156, 158, 162, 172, 186, 190, 196,
204–206, 211
locust pose, 67, 94, 106, 208
long deep breathing exercise, 36
looking under water exercise, 175
lotus pose, 40
love, 21, 26, 27, 34, 41, 57, 69
lower back, 35, 44, 53, 66, 72, 84, 124, 126,
128, 133, 146, 169, 176, 189, 194, 204, 211,
233
lung, 41, 99, 101, 118, 129, 145, 151, 155,
156, 162, 181, 190, 217
lymphatic system, 17

M

mantra, 38
master lock, 39, 40
master, 16, 19, 23, 32, 33
meditation, 19, 21, 22, 30, 32, 33, 37–45,
52, 54, 75, 83, 128, 132
meditation for exploring the cause of
disease, 44
meditation for internal nourishment, 41
menstrual problems, including cramps, 39,
42, 67, 142, 193–196
mental, 21, 24, 25, 30, 31, 37, 46, 61
metabolism, 38, 61, 178, 193
middle warmer—See triple warmer
migraine headaches, 142, 145, 176, See also
headaches
mind clearing pose, 88
mudras (hand positions), 22, 44
mulabandha—See root lock
mustard plaster, 194

N, O

neck, 39, 44, 53, 57, 71, 73, 135, 137, 142,
160, 167, 168, 171–177, 197–201, 223,
227, 233
neck lock, 39–40
nerves, 15, 17, 20, 31, 33, 35, 37, 39, 40,
46, 51, 52, 127, 142, 163, 160, 202–205,
223, 224, 228
nervous system, 17, 21, 29, 37, 38, 40, 61,
84, 125–127, 157, 188
nervousness, 126, 130, 153, 223, 233
nourishment, 17, 71, 134
oneness, 25, 26, 46
opening the bow, 103
organ meridians—See each individual organ
(lungs, large intestines, etc.)